Clinical Electrocardiography

4th Edition

Clinical Electrocardiography

4th Edition

B L Chia

MBBS, FRACP, FRCP (Edin), FAMS, FACC

EMERITUS PROFESSOR
DEPARTMENT OF MEDICINE
YONG LOO LIN SCHOOL OF MEDICINE
NATIONAL UNIVERSITY OF SINGAPORE
SINGAPORE

EMERITUS CONSULTANT
NATIONAL UNIVERSITY HEART CENTRE
SINGAPORE

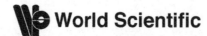

World Scientific

NEW JERSEY · LONDON · SINGAPORE · BEIJING · SHANGHAI · HONG KONG · TAIPEI · CHENNAI · TOKYO

Published by

World Scientific Publishing Co. Pte. Ltd.

5 Toh Tuck Link, Singapore 596224

USA office: 27 Warren Street, Suite 401-402, Hackensack, NJ 07601

UK office: 57 Shelton Street, Covent Garden, London WC2H 9HE

Library of Congress Cataloging-in-Publication Data
Chia, B. L. (Boon Lock), author.
Clinical electrocardiography / B. L. Chia. -- Fourth edition.
    p. ; cm.
   Includes index.
   ISBN 978-9814723251 (hardcover : alk. paper) -- ISBN 9814723258 (hardcover : alk. paper) --
   ISBN 978-9814723268 (paperback : alk. paper) -- ISBN 9814723266 (paperback : alk. paper)
   I. Title.
   [DNLM: 1. Electrocardiography--methods--Atlases. 2. Arrhythmias, Cardiac--diagnosis--Atlases. 3. Coronary
Artery Disease--diagnosis--Atlases. WG 17]
   RC683.5.E5
   616.1'207547--dc23
                                    2015029063

British Library Cataloguing-in-Publication Data
A catalogue record for this book is available from the British Library.

Disclaimer. Every effort and care has been taken to ensure accuracy of the information presented. However, the Publisher and author are not responsible for any errors or omissions. Neither the Publisher nor the author assume any liability for any injury or damage incurred directly or indirectly arising out of or related to any use of the material contained in this book. Application of the information in this book in a particular situation remains the professional responsibility of the practitioner.

Printed in Singapore

To

John, Cheryl, Emma and Peter

FOREWORD

For someone like myself who grew up learning electrocardiogram from the true master, Professor Boon-Lock Chia, this book surely is a must-read for anyone who is involved with cardiology care. This 4th Edition of Clinical Electrocardiography carries on the strengths of the previous editions in that it is an easy-to-read book, supplemented with simple explanations and illustrations that are relevant to daily clinical practice. The book rightly focuses on the two most common and important applications of ECG, which is in the diagnosis of acute myocardial infarction and cardiac arrhythmias. It is a book of reference for all levels of readers, from medical students to practising cardiologists.

Having known Prof Chia for the past 25 years through personal interaction, I can personally testify to his total commitment and lifelong dedication to the learning and teaching of the Art and Science of electrocardiography. This book is an extension of his continual work in ECG teaching. It showcases the best ECG tracings in his lifelong collection, with unique commentaries and insights arising from his wealth of personal clinical experience. His commitment in education is clearly depicted in the way that the ECGs are being presented – so clearly, precisely and in such an empowering manner. For Prof Chia, the book is truly a labour of love, and will be his lasting legacy.

Professor Huay-Cheem Tan
Senior Consultant and Director
National University Heart Centre, Singapore

Professor, Yong Loo Lin School of Medicine
National University of Singapore, Singapore

PREFACE

What a humbling experience it has been writing this new edition. Seventeen long years have slipped by since the 3rd Edition was published in 1998. During this very long period of time, cardiology and all its subspecialties, including electrocardiography, have advanced by leaps and bounds. Progress has been especially remarkable in the electrocardiographic diagnosis of acute myocardial infarction (STEMI) and the cardiac arrhythmias.

Five of the seven chapters in this 4th Edition have been extensively revised. In addition, nearly every ECG topic that is relevant and important to patient care has been included. One of the major strengths of the first three editions has been the quality of the ECG illustrations. In keeping with this tradition, the ECG illustrations in this fourth edition have been improved further, and out of the total 125 ECGs, 65 are new. Each ECG is crisp and clear and all the abnormalities are highlighted by either arrows or arrowheads for easy recognition and understanding. In addition, there are 17 figures/illustrations of which 11 are new; 4 coronary angiograms, all new; and 1 echocardiogram.

Books, monographs and scientific papers on electrocardiography abound and it would appear that there is little justification for yet another book on this subject. However, despite the voluminous publications, it is difficult to find books on electrocardiography which are short, simple, concise, accurate and relevant to patient care.

This book is the culmination of about 45 years of experience in the teaching of electrocardiography to coronary care unit nurses, medical undergraduates, postgraduates, residents and senior residents. As the title of the book implies, the approach to the subject has been entirely from the viewpoint of a clinician. Hence, theoretical considerations have been kept to a minimum and clinical-electrocardiogaphic correlations have been emphasized throughout the text.

Professor Boon-Lock Chia
2015

ACKNOWLEDGEMENTS

This 4th Edition could not have been written without the help, support, generosity and inspiration from my colleagues and friends at the Department of Cardiology, National University Heart Centre Singapore (NUHCS), with whom I have had the privilege and good fortune to work with over the past 20 years.

It gives me great pleasure to express my thanks and gratitude to the following: (1) Professor Huay-Cheem Tan, Director, NUHCS, an outstanding leader who so graciously agreed to write the Foreword to this 4th Edition. (2) The following Associate Professors and Senior Consultants: Tiong-Cheng Yeo, Head, Department of Cardiology NUHCS, Kian-Keong Poh, Post-graduate Medical Education Director, James Yip, Programme Director, Congenital and Structural Heart Disease, Adrian Low, Clinical Director, Cardiovascular Laboratory; and Mark Chan, Clinician Scientist, Cardiovascular Research Institute who so kindly read through the Chapter on Ischaemic Heart Disease and offered many important suggestions.

In addition, I would also like to thank the following: (1) Assistant Professor Swee-Chong Seow, Senior Consultant, Director, Cardiac Electrophysiology and Pacing and Director, Heart Rhythm Programme, who read through the Chapters on Cardiac Arrhythmias, Supraventricular Arrhythmias and Ventricular Arrhythmias and made major improvements in several areas. (2) Dr Wee-Siong Teo – eminent electrophysiologist at the National Heart Centre, Singapore and also at the Mount Elizabeth Medical Centre, Singapore – for our fruitful discussions and for his expert opinions on many issues pertaining to this book. I had the privilege and good fortune to have known and to have discussed ECG matters with Wee Siong since 1986. (3) Dr Swee-Guan Teo, Cardiologist at Raffles Hospital Singapore for his incredible skills in digitally printing some of the ECGs used in this book. (4) Ms Elisdawatinizam Mahat for her excellent editorial skills. (5) Ms Nanmullai Ramasamy for the digital graphics and (6) Ms Irene Chua for her clerical assistance.

Last but by no means least, I would like to express my sincere thanks and appreciation to Associate Professor Yean-Teng Lim, for his support and generosity when he was Chief, Cardiac Department (1999–2003) and Chairman Medical Board (1 January 2003–31 December 2005), both at the National University Hospital, Singapore.

Acknowledgements:

Dr Kit-Yee Chan for Fig. 5.17, Dr Bernard Ee for Figs. 2.9, 7.8 and 7.12, the late Dr A Johan for Fig. 5.6, Dr Chee-Choong Koo for Fig. 7.11, and Associate Professor Swee-Chye Quek for Fig. 3.26, The Managing Editor of Asian Medical News and the Editor of PULSE for permission to reproduce several of the ECG quizzes which I have previously published, The Editor of the *Singapore Medical Journal* for permission to reproduce from my previous publications Figs. 2.27, 5.18 and 5.19 and The Editor-in-Chief, *The Canadian Journal of Cardiology* for permission to reproduce from my previous publication Fig. 7.3.

Professor Boon-Lock Chia
2015

CONTENTS

Foreword   vii

Preface   ix

Acknowledgements   xi

1. The Normal Electrocardiogram   1

2. Ischaemic Heart Disease   15

3. Miscellaneous Conditions   47

4. Cardiac Arrhythmias   73

5. Supraventricular Arrhythmias   77

6. Ventricular Arrhythmias   97

7. Bundle Branch Block, Hemiblock and Atrioventricular (AV) Block   117

Index   129

CHAPTER 1

THE NORMAL ELECTROCARDIOGRAM

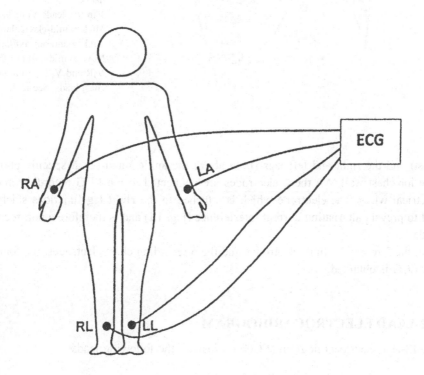

Fig. 1.1 Electrodes are attached to the body surface to record an ECG. The right leg electrode functions solely as a ground to prevent alternating current interference and is a non-recording electrode. (Abbreviations: RA = right arm, LA = left arm, RL = right leg, LL = left leg).

An electrocardiogram or ECG is the recording of the electrical activity generated by the cells of the heart which reaches the surface of the body. This is achieved by attaching electrodes which are simply disposable paste-on disks or metal plates used to detect the electrical currents of the heart. These electrodes are placed on (1) the limbs – the right and left arms (both above

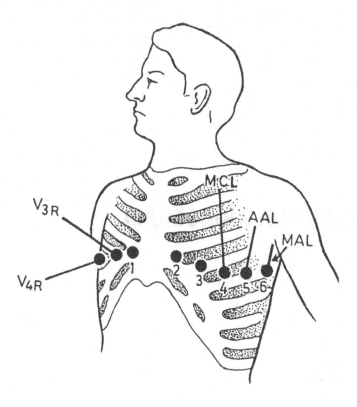

Fig. 1.2 Diagram showing the positions of the electrode when recording the different left and right-sided chest leads.

1 to 6 = leads V_1 to V_6.

MCL = mid-clavicular line,

AAL = anterior axillary line,

MAL = mid-axillary line,

V_3R and V_4R = right-sided chest leads. See text.

the wrist) and the right and left legs (both above the ankles) and (2) at specific points on the anterior chest wall. All these electrodes are connected to the ECG recording machine via electrical wires. The electrode which is attached to the **right leg** functions solely as a **ground** to prevent alternating current interference (Fig. 1.1) and is therefore a non-recording electrode.

From the 3 recording limb electrodes and the 6 recording chest electrodes, the following 12-lead ECG is obtained.

The 12-LEAD ELECTROCARDIOGRAM

The 12-lead electrocardiogram (ECG) consists of the following leads

(1) Six Limb (Extremity) Leads

The six limb leads (which are all in the **frontal plane**) consist of 3 **bipolar leads** – lead I *(between the right and left arm)*, lead II *(between the right arm and the left leg)*, lead III *(between the left arm and the left leg)*, and 3 **augmented unipolar leads** – leads aVR *(right arm)*, aVL *(left arm)* and aVF *(left leg) (a = augmented)*.

(2) Six Unipolar Chest Leads

These are designated as V leads. There are six V leads **(from V_1 to V_6)** depending on where the electrode is placed on the chest (Fig. 1.2). Lead V_1 is recorded with the electrode on the fourth intercostal space just to the right of the sternum, and lead V_2 on the fourth intercostal space just to the left of the sternum. Lead V_3 is recorded at a position exactly mid-way between leads V_2 and V_4. Lead V_4 is recorded on the fifth left intercostal space in the mid-clavicular line. Leads V_5 and V_6 are recorded at the same horizontal level as lead V_4, with lead V_5 in the left anterior axillary line and lead V_6 in the left mid-axillary line.

Apart from the above conventional 12 leads, other leads such as **right-sided chest leads** V_3R, V_4R, V_5R and V_6R are recorded in positions which correspond to leads V_3, V_4, V_5 and V_6 respectively, except that the electrodes are now placed on the right side of the chest instead of on the left. These leads (especially lead V_4R) are particularly useful for the diagnosis of right ventricular infarction.

Recently, **leads V_7, V_8 and V_9** have been reported to be valuable in the diagnosis of posterior myocardial infarction. These 3 leads are recorded at the same horizontal level as lead V_6, with the electrode being placed in the left posterior axilliary line for lead V_7, left mid-scapular line for lead V_8 and at the left border of the spine for lead V_9. Although useful, they have not proven to be popular and are not done frequently.

CALCULATION OF HEART RATE

There are 2 methods of calculating the heart rate: **(1) Box Counting Method (2) QRS Counting Method**.

Box Counting Method

The ECG is normally recorded at a speed of **25 mm/sec**. The horizontal distance between 1 **large box** on the ECG paper recorded at this speed represents 0.20 sec. Since this distance spans the length of 5 small boxes, each **small box** therefore represents **0.04 sec**.

A simple way to calculate the heart rate is to **divide 300 by the number of large boxes between 2 consecutive beats** if the rhythm is regular. For example, the following are the heart rates corresponding to the number of large boxes in between 2 consecutive beats.

Heart Rate	Number of Large Boxes between 2 Consecutive Beats
300	1 (300/1)
150	2 (300/2)
100	3 (300/3)
75	4 (300/4)
60	5 (300/5)
50	6 (300/6)
43	7 (300/7)
38	8 (300/8)

The rationale for the above calculation is as follows. There are 300 fifths of a second in 1 minute (5 × 60). One fifth of a second (i.e. 0.20 sec) is represented by 1 large box. Therefore, the heart rate is conveniently calculated by dividing 300 by the number of large boxes between 2 consecutive beats. The Box Counting Method is accurate when the rhythm is regular, but inaccurate when it is irregular.

QRS Counting Method

This method for counting an average heart rate is accurate when the rhythm is regular or irregular (e.g. atrial fibrillation). At the normal recording speed of 25 mm/sec, the **recording time** of most 12-lead ECG recordings is **10 seconds** (Fig. 1.3). Simply counting the number of QRS complexes within this 10 second interval and **multiplying it by 6** will give you the average heart rate in beats/min.

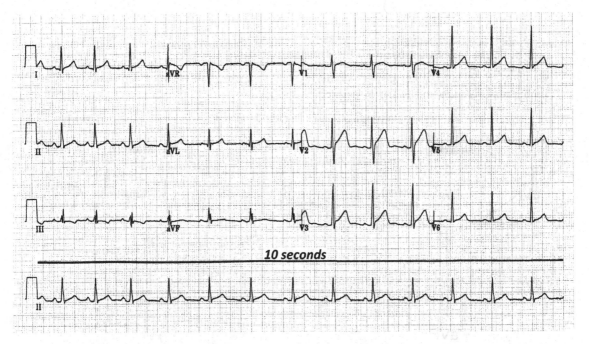

Fig. 1.3 Calculation of heart rate by **QRS counting method**. The number of QRS complexes in 10 sec is 13. Therefore the heart rate is 13 × 6 = 78 beats per minute. Using the **Box counting method** – the number of large boxes between 2 consecutive beats is 4. Therefore the heart rate is 300 ÷ 4 = 75 beats per minute. The extreme left shows **ECG calibration** – 1 millivolt signal = 10 mm vertical amplitude (see text).

Calculating QRS Axis

The **QRS axis** is defined as the **mean QRS vector in the frontal plane**. It is determined using the hexaxial reference system which is described below.

The **Einthoven's equilateral triangle** is formed by leads I, II and III (Fig. 1.4). A **triaxial reference system** is obtained by redrawing the Einthoven's triangle so that leads I, II and III intersect at a common central point (Fig. 1.4). This is done simply by sliding lead I downwards, lead II to the right and lead III to the left.

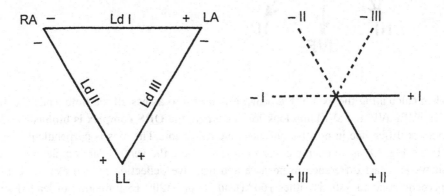

Fig. 1.4 (Left hand panel) Einthoven's equilateral triangle. (Right hand panel) Converting Einthoven's equilateral triangle to a triaxial reference system. (Abbreviations: RA = right arm, LA = left arm, LL = left leg, Ld I = lead I, Ld II = lead II, Ld III = lead III) (see text).

A similar triaxial reference system can be obtained, this time by using the 3 augmented unipolar leads aVR, aVL and aVF (Fig. 1.5). Finally, the 2 triaxial reference systems can be combined to obtain the **hexaxial reference system** that shows the relationship of all the 6 limb leads (Figs. 1.6 and 1.7).

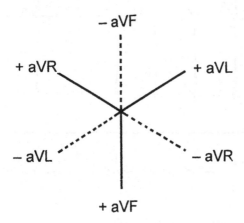

Fig. 1.5 Triaxial reference system obtained from leads aVR, aVL and aVF (see text).

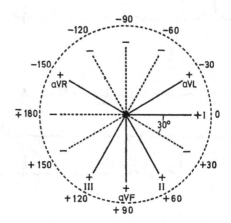

Fig. 1.6 Hexaxial reference system obtained from the previous 2 triaxial reference systems (see text).

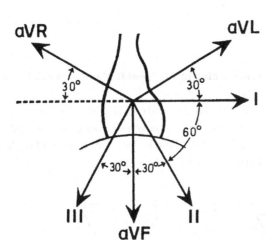

Fig. 1.7 Hexaxial reference system diagram that is used clinically.

When calculating the axis of the heart, it is useful to assess all the limb leads (i.e. leads I, II, III, aVR, aVL and aVF) and look for one where the **QRS complex is biphasic** and has the smallest difference in positive and negative deflection. The axis is perpendicular to this lead. Using Fig. 1.8 as an example, the limb lead where the ventricular complex is biphasic and shows the least difference in positive and negative deflection is lead aVL (−30°). The axis perpendicular to −30° is either +60° (lead II) or −120°. Examination of lead II shows that the QRS complex is upright and therefore the axis must be directed towards the positive pole of this lead (i.e. the axis is +60°). If the axis is −120°, the QRS complex in lead II will be negative.

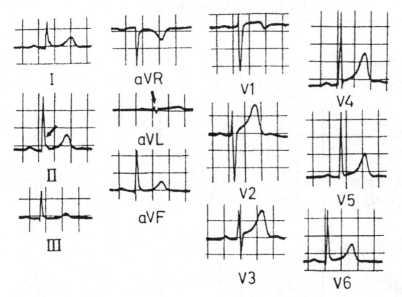

Fig. 1.8 12-lead ECG from a normal young man. This same ECG is repeated in Fig. 3.1 in page 47. The limb lead where the ventricular complex is biphasic and has the smallest difference in positive and negative deflection is lead aVL (−30°) [arrow]. The axis perpendicular to −30° is either +60° or −120°. Since lead II [arrow] shows that the QRS is upright, the axis must be around +60° (see text).

In clinical practice, precise calculation of the QRS axis is not as important as knowing whether it is normal, left axis deviation or right axis deviation. This recognition can be easily achieved just by looking at the QRS complexes in **leads I and II**. If the QRS is predominantly positive in leads I and II the axis is normal. If it is positive in lead I and negative in lead II, left axis deviation is present. Lastly, if it is negative in lead I and positive in lead II, right axis deviation is present (Fig. 1.9).

The **normal axis** is between −30° to +90°. **Left axis deviation** is defined as an axis that is −30° to −90° and **right axis deviation** as an axis that is +90° to +180°. When the axis is between −90° and +180° (i.e. upper right quadrant), the axis is termed **"indeterminate"**.

	Lead I	Lead II
Normal Axis		
Left Axis Deviation		
Right Axis Deviation		

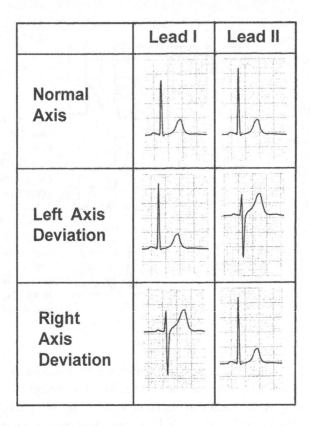

Fig. 1.9 Simple method for determining whether the QRS axis is normal or whether there is left or right axis deviation (see text).

COMPLEXES, SEGMENTS and TIME INTERVALS (Figs. 1.10, 1.11 and 1.12)

> **In this book, all the 12-lead ECGs and the cardiac rhythm strips are recorded at 25 mm/sec** (as in normal clinical practice). **Therefore, 1 small box horizontally = 0.04 sec and 1 big box = 0.20 sec.** Likewise, the **ECG is calibrated so that 1 millivolt signal produces a vertical deflection of 10 mm amplitude** (as in normal clinical practice).

P Wave

The P wave represents atrial depolarization which proceeds downwards anterogradely from the sinoatrial node. It is normally upright in leads I, II, aVF and the left praecordial leads V_4 to V_6, inverted in lead aVR, and biphasic in lead V_1. The polarity of the P wave in all the other leads is variable. The P wave should be less than 0.12 sec in duration and less than 2.5 mm in height in leads II, III and aVF and less than 1.5 mm in leads V_1 or V_2.

PR Segment

The PR segment is the portion between the end of the P wave and the beginning of the QRS complex.

P-QRS-T

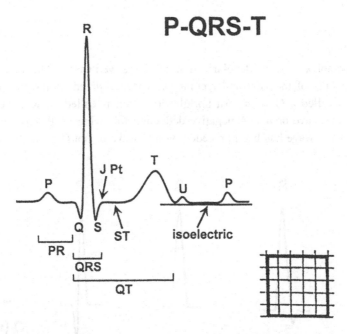

Fig. 1.10 Diagram showing the various ECG complexes, segments and time intervals (see text. J Pt = J point. isoelectric = isoelectric line).

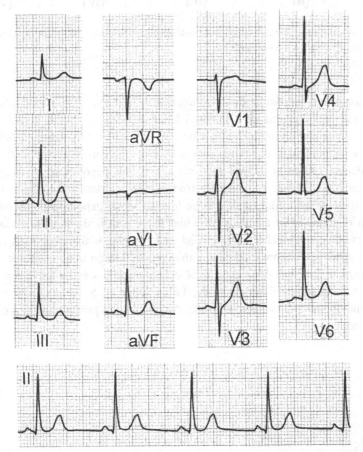

Fig. 1.11 Normal 12-lead ECG from a 70-year-old man (see text).

QRS Complex

The QRS complex reflects depolarization of the 2 ventricles. The nomenclature of the various segments of the ventricular complex is standardized. If the first deflection is downwards, it is called a **Q** wave. An upright deflection is called an **R** wave, whether it is preceded by a Q wave or not. A negative deflection following an R wave is called an **S** wave, whether the R wave has been preceded by a Q wave or not (Fig. 1.12).

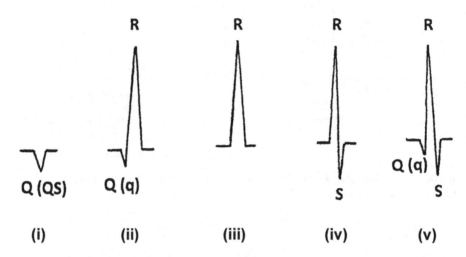

Fig. 1.12 Nomenclature of the various segments of the ventricular complex: (i) Q wave (ii, iii) R wave (iv, v) S wave (see text).

Depolarization of the ventricular myocardium begins in the septum, where it takes place in a left to right direction (sequence 1 in Fig. 1.13). Following this, both the left and right ventricles are depolarized simultaneously. However, since the left ventricle has a much larger physical and electrical mass, ventricular depolarization can be conveniently regarded electrically as depolarization of the left ventricle alone. This depolarization proceeds from right to left (sequence 2 in Fig. 1.13). An electrode which is orientated to the left ventricle (e.g. lead V_5) will show an initial small q wave (due to septal depolarization moving away from the electrode), followed by a large R wave (due to the ventricular depolarization moving towards the electrode). A typical left praecordial lead complex is therefore a qR complex.

The same electrical events are recorded in an opposite fashion in an electrode orientated to the right ventricle (e.g. lead V_1). The initial deflection is a small r wave due to septal depolarization moving towards the electrode, followed by an S wave due to ventricular depolarization moving away from the electrode. A typical right praecordial lead complex is therefore an rS complex (Fig. 1.13).

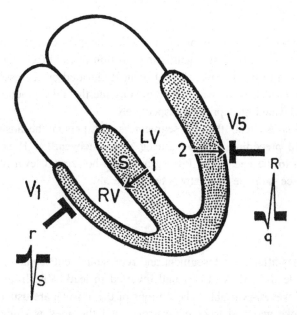

Fig. 1.13 Diagram showing normal sequence of ventricular depolarization and the ventricular complexes in V_1 and V_5. S = septum, RV = right ventricle, LV = left ventricle (see text).

In the praecordial leads, rS complexes are seen in leads V_1 and V_2 and qR complexes in leads V_4 to V_6. There is gradual increase in the height of the r wave and a corresponding decrease in depth of the S wave from leads V_1 to V_3. In lead **V_3** or **V_4** which represents the **transitional zone**, the height of the R wave and the depth of the S wave are approximately equal. In the limb leads, the ventricular complexes may show either a left or a right praecordial lead pattern. The only exception is **lead aVR**, where the ventricular complex normally shows a negative deflection in the form of either a **Qr complex** (a prominent Q wave followed by a small r wave), an **rS complex** (a small r wave followed by a deep S wave) or a **QS complex** (only 1 prominent Q wave). The **P wave and T wave** are normally **inverted in lead aVR**.

Normally, the 2 ventricles are depolarized simultaneously, resulting in a narrow QRS complex which is 0.05 to 0.10 second in duration. In ventricular ectopic beats, bundle branch block, supraventricular ectopic beats with aberrant ventricular conduction, or Preexcitation (Wolff-Parkinson-White ECG pattern) the 2 ventricles are depolarized non-simultaneously, resulting in a QRS complex that is widened to ≥ 0.12 second.

There is a wide variation in the normal voltage/amplitude of the QRS complex. It is significantly greater in men compared to women. The amplitude increases until the age of about 30 years and then starts decreasing gradually. The generally accepted upper limit for the R wave in lead V_5/V_6 is about 26 mm. However, amplitudes greater than this are commonly present in thin, normal, young individuals, in athletes and in those whose ECG show the Early Repolarization Pattern (see Chapter 3).

ST Segment

The **J point** is defined as the junction of the end of the QRS complex and the beginning of the ST segment. Hence, the ST segment is that portion of the ECG that is between the J point and the beginning of the T wave. If the J point is elevated or depressed with reference to the isoelectric line (which is the baseline formed by the the TP segment), the ST segment is considered to be elevated or depressed respectively.

During exercise stress test, the TP segment is not present because the P wave is superimposed on the preceding T wave during sinus tachycardia. Hence the J point is measured in relation to the end of the PR segment, the horizontal level of which becomes the isoelectric line (see exercise ECG stress test, page 38).

T Wave

The T wave comes after the ST segment and represents ventricular repolarization. It is normally upright in leads I, II, V_3 to V_6 and inverted in lead aVR. In all the other leads, the polarity of the T wave is variable. The 2 limbs of the T wave are usually asymmetrical, with a slower upstroke and a sharper downstroke, and the apex is slightly rounded. The amplitude of the T wave, like that of the QRS complex, has wide normal limits. However, it tends to diminish with age and is smaller in females. The upper limit of the T wave in all the limb leads is < 6 mm. In the praecordial leads in males, it may reach ≥ 10 mm, but in females it is seldom > 8 mm. However, very tall T waves are frequently seen in the Early Repolarization Pattern, even though there is no cardiac or other disease.

U Wave

The U wave follows the T wave. The genesis of the U wave is unclear but one of the theories is tardy repolarization of the subendocardial Purkinje fibres. It is normally of low amplitude, with many ECGs having no discernable U wave and has the same polarity as the T wave. It is usually most prominent in leads V_2 to V_4 and generally does not exceed 2 mm or one quarter of the height of the preceding T wave (Fig. 1.10).

INTERVALS

PR Interval

The PR interval is measured from the onset of the P wave to the beginning of the QRS or rS complex. It represents the time taken for the sinus impulse to travel across the atria, down the atrioventricular (AV) node, bundle of His, bundle branches, Purkinje fibres and finally to the ventricular myocardium of both ventricles. It is normally 0.12 to 0.20 sec in duration.

QT Interval

The QT interval is measured from the onset of the QRS complex to the end of the T wave. As a general rule, the QT interval should not be longer than half of the interval between adjacent R waves (R-R interval). Since the normal QT interval varies with the heart rate, the QTc or the corrected QT interval is used clinically instead of the QT interval. The QTc is calculated from the QT interval and the heart rate using the Bazett formula: QTc = QT interval divided by the square root of the R-R interval measured in seconds. Many investigators consider the upper limit of normal for QTc for both genders to be 0.44 sec. However, some have suggested higher values and the following Bazett-corrected QTc values for diagnosing QT prolongation: in adult males < 0.43 sec (normal), 0.43 to 0.45 sec (borderline) and > 0.45 sec (prolonged) and in adult females < 0.45 sec (normal), 0.45 to 0.47 sec (borderline) and > 0.47 sec (prolonged).

CHAPTER 2

ISCHAEMIC HEART DISEASE

The two major clinical applications of electrocardiography are the diagnosis of: (1) acute myocardial infarction and other types of myocardial ischaemia and (2) cardiac arrhythmias. The birth of electrocardiography more than 10 decades ago opened a new dimension in the study of the heart, by allowing the cardiac electrical currents (voltages, potentials) to be clinically recorded for the first time. This heralded a new era in the diagnosis and treatment of coronary artery disease and cardiac arrhythmias.

Despite the introduction in recent years of many new investigative techniques such as echocardiography, myocardial perfusion imaging, cardiac magnetic resonance imaging, computed tomography coronary angiography and invasive coronary angiography, the electrocardiogram today still retains its pivotal role in the evaluation of acute myocardial infarction, chiefly because it is useful, very simple to perform, noninvasive and inexpensive.

In this chapter, various ECG patterns of acute myocardial infarction (ST elevation myocardial infarction [STEMI] and non-ST elevation myocardial infarction [NSTEMI]) and other ischaemic heart disease, and pitfalls in their diagnoses will be discussed. The many problems that are frequently encountered in the ECG evaluation of non-ischaemic ST segment elevation and depression and their differentiation from STEMI and NSTEMI will be discussed in the next chapter, which deals with ECG abnormalities seen in miscellaneous conditions.

PRESENTATION OF ISCHAEMIC HEART DISEASE

Coronary artery disease may present in several different ways. A significant number of individuals who suffer from this disease have no symptoms at all even though the disease is severe. They have what is known as **silent myocardial ischaemia**. Others however may manifest with **acute transmural myocardial infarction (ST elevation myocardial infarction [STEMI]) or acute subendocardial myocardial infarction (non-ST elevation myocardial infarction [NSTEMI]), stable and unstable angina pectoris, sudden cardiac death and heart failure**.

Whenever an ECG is recorded in a patient who is suspected of having ischaemic heart disease, the following questions should be routinely asked:

(1) Is the ECG normal or abnormal?
(2) If it is abnormal, do the abnormalities indicate myocardial infarction, angina pectoris or some other condition?
(3) If the ECG is indicative of myocardial infarction, do the changes suggest an acute or a chronic myocardial infarction?

These questions are of obvious importance, because the clinical significance in terms of urgency of management in patients suffering from acute myocardial infarction versus patients suffering from stable angina pectoris or chronic ischaemic heart disease is completely different.

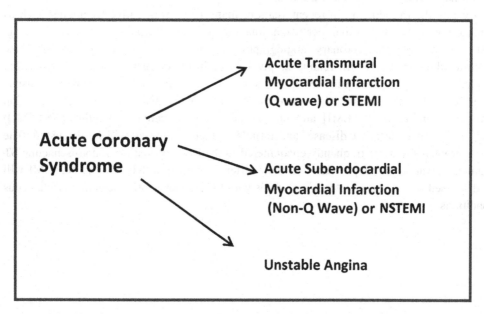

Fig. 2.1 Classification of acute coronary syndrome. (Abbreviations: STEMI = ST elevation myocardial infarction. NSTEMI = non-ST elevation myocardial infarction).

ACUTE MYOCARDIAL INFARCTION

In 2011, there were more than 2 thousand cases of STEMI in Singapore. In that year, the total number of Singapore residents was 3.8 million. **Early diagnosis** of acute myocardial infarction is of crucial importance because: (1) Mortality is highest in the first few hours and (2) Thrombolytic therapy or percutaneous coronary intervention, very often with stenting, is most effective if they are administered early after the onset of infarction.

The 4 principal parameters for evaluation are:
(1) Clinical history and patient's cardiovascular risk profile
(2) Physical examination
(3) 12-lead ECG
(4) Serum biomarkers of acute myocardial infarction such as creatinine phosphokinase **(CK)**, CKMB fraction **(CKMB)** and **troponin**.

Since the levels of the serum biomarkers of acute myocardial infarction may not be significantly elevated in the first few hours after the onset of the infarction, early diagnosis must frequently depend on the clinical history and the ECG findings.

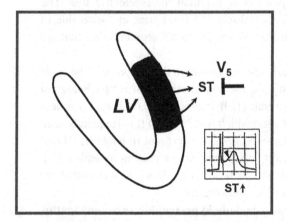 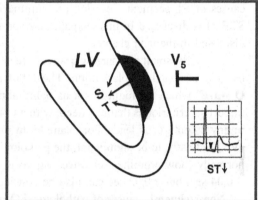

Fig. 2.2   With acute transmural (epicardial) ischaemia (left hand panel), the ST segment vector is deviated outwards. An overlying lead (V_5) will record an ST segment elevation. In the presence of acute subendocardial ischaemia (right hand panel), the ST segment vector is deviated inwards. An overlying lead (V_5) will record ST segment depression. (Abbreviation: LV = left ventricle).

Acute myocardial infarction is very often due to a thrombus which is superimposed on a ruptured atherosclerotic plaque, obstructing coronary blood flow. If the obstruction is total, **transmural myocardial infarction**, where the whole thickness of the myocardium is involved, will occur. An ECG lead which is placed over the site of the infarction ("indicative changes") shows ST segment elevation – hence the terminology of "ST Elevation Myocardial Infarction" or **STEMI** (Fig. 2.2). In contrast, a subtotal occlusion of the coronary artery will result in a **subendocardial myocardial infarction** and here, the ST segment is depressed resulting in the terminology of "non-ST Elevation Myocardial Infarction" or **NSTEMI**. ST segment depression is also the signature ECG abnormality in **unstable angina** and **stable angina pectoris**.

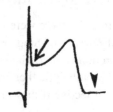

Causes of ST Segment Elevation

- STEMI
- Other Causes
  - "Normal male pattern" · Acute pericarditis
  - Early repolarization pattern
  - Type 1 Brugada pattern
  - Acute pulmonary embolism
  - Left bundle branch block
  - Myocardial Disease
    - *(i) Left ventricular hypertrophy*
    - *(ii) Takotsubo cardiomyopathy*

Arrow indicates J point / ST segment elevation
Arrowhead indicates isoelectric line

Table 1. Causes of ST Segment Elevation

ST segment elevation occurs when the J point is higher than the isoelectric line. The causes of ST segment elevation are summarized in Table 1. ST segment elevation due to STEMI is discussed in this chapter, and non-ischaemic causes of ST segment elevation are discussed in the next chapter.

Normally, small and narrow q waves are nearly always present in the left praecordial leads because of septal depolarization. The following are the characteristics of a **"pathological Q wave"** which distinguishes it as being abnormal: (1) It is broad ($\geq$ 0.04 sec). (2) A less important criterion is that it is deep, with a Q/R ratio which is $\geq$ 25%. (3) It is frequently seen in any 2 contiguous leads. For example, in inferior STEMI, it is present in leads II, III and aVF. (4) Lastly, to be significant, the pathological Q wave must not be present in leads which normally show prominent Q waves e.g. aVR & V_1. (5) In leads V_2 & V_3, Q waves that are < 0.04 sec, but $\geq$ 0.02 sec can also be considered as pathological.

Non-ischaemic causes of pathological Q waves **include hypertrophic cardiomyopathy, dilated cardiomyopathy and acute pulmonary embolism.**

EVOLUTIONARY ECG PATTERN of STEMI

Figure 2.3 shows the evolutionary ECG pattern of acute transmural myocardial infarction or STEMI. In the **"hyperacute phase"** (i.e. during the first few hours), the ST segments are elevated with a slope which is either concave or straight upwards. The T waves are frequently tall. ST segments in leads overlying normal myocardium which are opposite to the infarct site will show **"reciprocal" ST segment depression** (B in Fig. 2.3 and Fig. 2.4). In this phase of acute myocardial infarction, pathological Q waves and T wave inversion are not seen. It is important to note that even though the clinical presentation is typical for STEMI, the initial ECG in the hyperacute phase may show either nonspecific abnormalities or it may even be normal. In this situation, it is important to repeat the 12-lead ECG recording every 15 minutes, because serial ECGs will frequently show diagnostic STEMI changes (Fig. 2.7). The current treatment of STEMI is either **thrombolytic therapy** or, preferably if it is available, **percutaneous coronary intervention (PCI) with stenting.**

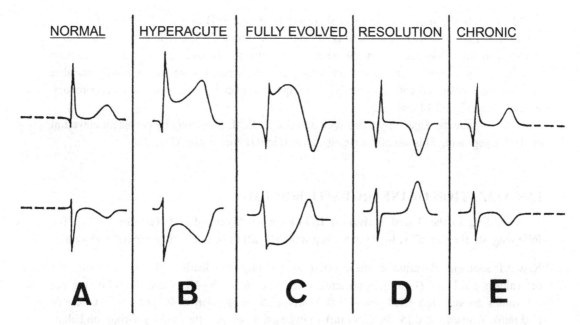

NORMAL	HYPERACUTE	FULLY EVOLVED	RESOLUTION	CHRONIC

A   B   C   D   E

Fig.2.3 Diagram showing the ECG changes in transmural myocardial infarction or STEMI. Top panel shows the ECG changes in the leads facing the infarct site (i.e. "indicative changes"). Bottom panel shows the ECG changes in the leads facing the opposite normal myocardium (i.e. "reciprocal changes").

Generally, within 24 hours of the onset of acute myocardial infarction, the ST segment elevation decreases and pathological Q waves start to develop. The elevated ST segments, unlike those seen in the "hyperacute phase", are now convex upwards. Later in this phase which is called **"the fully evolved phase"**, deep and symmetrically inverted T waves are seen (C in Fig. 2.3 and Fig. 2.5).

Following the "fully evolved phase", the ECG begins to show the **"resolution phase"**. During this period, the ST segments fall to the isoelectric line, but the inverted T waves and the pathological Q waves remain (D in Fig. 2.3). Still later, in the **"chronic phase"** the T waves become upright and all that remains are the pathological Q waves (E in Fig. 2.3 and Fig. 2.6). The terms "chronic phase" of myocardial infarction and "old myocardial infarction" are frequently used synonymously. In some patients, the pathological Q waves become less prominent or may even disappear completely after several months or years. With the passage of time, small r waves are occasionally resurrected in leads which originally showed pathological Q waves. If this occurs in leads V_1 to V_3, the height of the r waves may not increase progressively as in the normal ECG. This phenomenon is referred to as **"poor r wave progression"**, which often indicates an old anterior infarction. However, this abnormality may also be seen in left ventricular hypertrophy or dilated cardiomyopathy (Fig. 3.14).

To illustrate the sequence, an ECG abnormality shown in B in Fig. 2.2 indicates a recent myocardial infarction perhaps a few hours old, in C about 24 hours later in time, in D a few days to weeks old and in E a few weeks to months old. However, it is important to note that the time sequence of all these evolutionary changes described above are highly variable and may be accelerated with thrombolytic therapy or especially after percutaneous coronary intervention (Figs. 2.14 and 2.15).

In some patients, especially those with anterior STEMI, there may be persistent elevation of the ST segment. This usually suggests a **ventricular aneurysm** (Fig. 2.8).

LOCALIZATION OF INFARCT SITE in STEMI

According to the **Third Universal Definition of Myocardial Infarction (2012),** the following are the **cut off values for ST segment elevation in acute myocardial ischaemia**:

New ST segment elevation at the J point in 2 contiguous leads with the following cut off values: ≥ 0.1 mV (1 mm) in all leads other than leads V_2-V_3 where the following cut off values apply: Men < 40 yrs $- \geq 0.25$ mV (2.5 mm); Men ≥ 40 years $- \geq 0.20$ mV (2.0 mm). Women $- \geq 0.15$ mV (1.5 mm). (Thygesen K. et al. – the Writing Group on behalf of the Joint European Society of Cardiology/American College of Cardiology Foundation/American Heart Association/World Heart Federation Task Force for the Universal Definition of Myocardial Infarction. Third Universal Definition of Myocardial Infarction. Circulation 2012; 126: 2020).

In cases of STEMI, **reciprocal ST segment depression**, which is an electrical phenomenon that is not evidence of additional myocardial ischaemia, is very frequently seen. None of the chest or V leads which are all in the horizontal plane are reciprocal to any of the limb leads which are all in the frontal plane. Therefore, reciprocal ST segment depression is essentially a limb lead phenomenon, except for reciprocal ST segment depression in leads V_1, V_2 and V_3 resulting from ST segment elevation in leads V_7, V_8 and V_9 in posterior STEMI. To show reciprocal depression, the 2 involved leads must be at least > 90 degrees apart. In inferior STEMI, ST segment elevation is almost always seen in leads II, III and aVF and obligatory reciprocal ST segment depression is seen in leads I and aVL. Similarly, in anterior STEMI, ST segment elevation is seen in leads V_1/V_2 to V_5/V_6 as well as in leads I and aVL. It is the elevation in leads I and aVL that causes obligatory reciprocal ST segment depression in leads II, III and aVF. In a minority of cases of anterior STEMI, ST segment elevation is seen only in leads V_1/V_2 to V_5/V_6 and not in leads I and aVL. In such patients, no reciprocal ST segment depression is seen.

Finally, non-ischaemic ST segment elevation (e.g acute pulmonary embolism), occurring in any of the limb leads, can also cause obligatory reciprocal ST segment depression. Therefore, it is important to know that reciprocal ST segment depression is not unique to STEMI alone.

The incidence of anterior STEMI and inferior STEMI is approximately equal. The presence of ST segment elevation in certain leads suggests that STEMI has occurred in specific sites of the heart. For example, in **anterior STEMI**, ST segment elevation in leads V_1 to V_4 indicates anteroseptal/apical infarction, in leads V_5, V_6 anterolateral and leads I and aVL high lateral infarction of the **left ventricle**. In **inferior STEMI**, ST segment elevation in leads II, III, aVF indicates inferior infarction of the **left ventricle**. The culprit artery in anterior STEMI is most frequently the left anterior descending artery and very rarely the left main coronary artery. The culprit artery in inferior STEMI is the right coronary artery in about 80 to 90% of cases and the left circumflex artery in about 10 to 20% of cases.

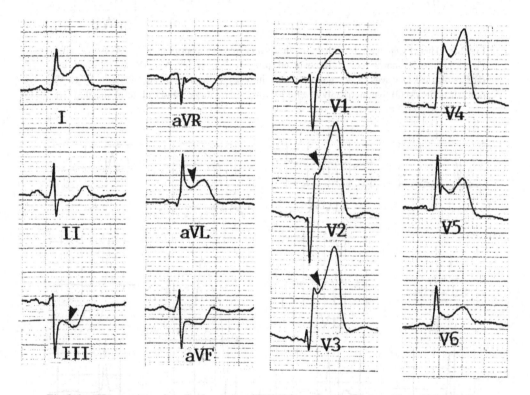

Fig. 2.4 "Hyperacute phase" of anterior STEMI in a 51-year-old man. Note: (1) Markedly elevated ST segments (concave upwards) in V_2 to V_6, I and aVL (arrowheads in V_2, V_3 and aVL) merging with tall T waves in V_2 to V_4 (ST elevation and T wave amplitude in V_2 = 10 mm and 20 mm respectively). (2) Reciprocal ST segment depression in II, III and aVF (arrowhead in III). Intravenous streptokinase therapy was given. Subsequent coronary angiography revealed a 90% stenosis of the proximal left anterior descending artery. (Reproduced with permission. Poh KK, HC Tan, Teo SG. ECG ST segment elevation in patients with chest pain. Sing Med J 2011; 52(1): 3 [with adaptation]).

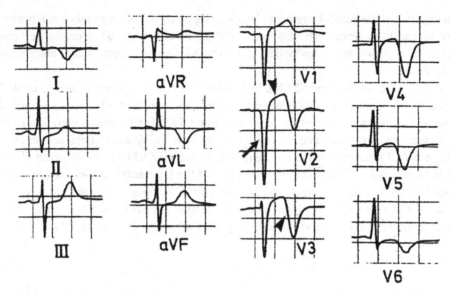

Fig. 2.5 This ECG was recorded in the same patient approximately 24 hours after Fig. 2.4. It now shows the **"fully evolved phase" of anterior STEMI** as reflected by: (1) Pathological Q waves in V_1 and V_2 (arrow in V_2) (2) Elevated ST segments in V_1 to V_3 (arrowhead in V_2) (3) Symmetrically inverted T waves in V_2 to V_6, I and aVL (arrowhead in V_3).

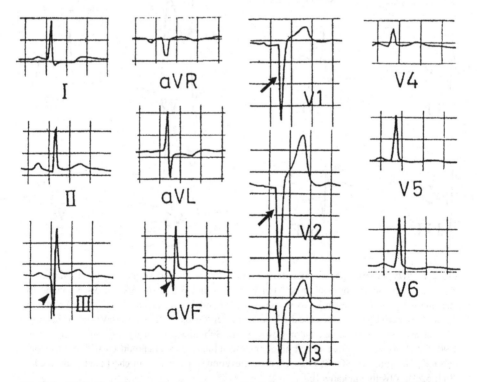

Fig. 2.6 ECG of a 70-year-old man showing the **"chronic phase" of inferior STEMI** as reflected by pathological Q waves in leads III and aVF (arrowheads). These Q waves are also seen in V_1 and V_2 (arrows). However since ST elevation is also seen in these 2 leads, the age of the anterior STEMI is uncertain.

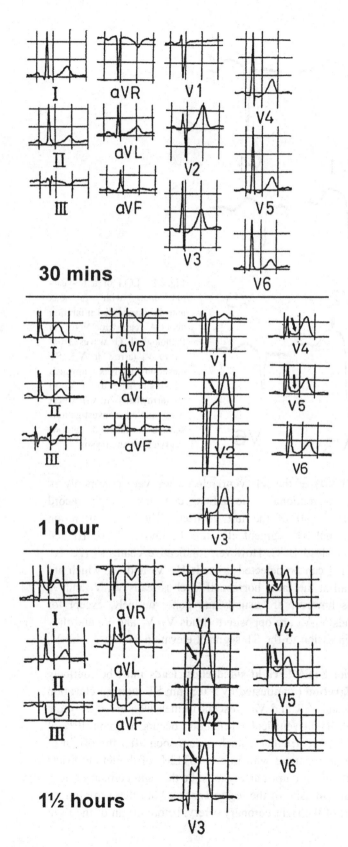

30 mins

1 hour

1½ hours

Fig. 2.7 shows 3 sequential ECGs' of a 55-year-old man who was strongly suspected of having STEMI. The first ECG (upper panel) recorded 30 minutes after the onset of chest pain was normal. The second ECG (middle panel) recorded 1 hour after the onset of chest pain showed subtle but significant ECG changes. Mild ST segment elevation has occurred in V_2 to V_6 and aVL (arrows in V_4, V_5 and aVL). There is reciprocal ST depression in III (arrow). The T wave in V_2 has become much taller (arrow). The third ECG (bottom panel) recorded one and a half hours after the onset of chest pain showed classical changes of anterior STEMI – marked ST elevation in V_2 to V_5, I and aVL (arrows) with reciprocal ST depression in III and aVF. Therefore, it is important to repeat the 12-lead ECG at 15 minute intervals if the patient is clinically diagnosed as having STEMI but the first ECG shows either non-diagnostic changes or is normal.

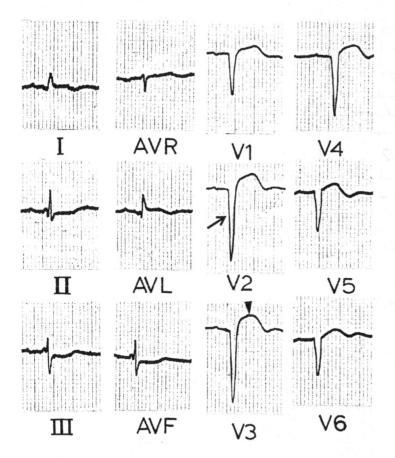

Fig. 2.8 ECG of a 62-year-old man with previous anterior myocardial infarction about 4 years ago. Note: (1) Pathological Q waves from V_1 to V_4 (arrow in V_2). ST elevation (convex upwards and dome shaped) in V_1 to V_4 (arrowhead in V_3). Chest X-ray and other investigations showed a calcified anterior **ventricular aneurysm**.

Acute **posterior infarction (STEMI)** of the **left ventricle** occurs very commonly in patients with inferior STEMI. The conventional 12-lead ECG does not directly record electrical currents from the posterior wall of the left ventricle. Therefore, infarction at this site does not manifest additional ST segment elevation beyond leads II, III and aVF due to inferior STEMI in the 12-lead ECG. However, "indicative changes" (i.e. ST segment elevation) of posterior STEMI can be detected in leads V_7, V_8 and V_9, which are placed on the left posterior chest wall at the same horizontal level as leads V_4, V_5 and V_6 (Fig. 2.10). These 3 posterior leads however are usually not done routinely, except for research purposes. Nevertheless, leads V_1-V_3 are opposite to leads V_7, V_8 and V_9 and they will show reciprocal ST segment depression to the ST segment elevation in V_7, V_8 and V_9 in posterior STEMI.

If the 12-lead ECG shows inferior STEMI, **right-sided chest leads** must be routinely done to detect **right ventricular infarction** (manifested by > 0.5 mm ST segment elevation especially in lead V_4R but also in leads V_5R and V_6R, except in men who are < 30 years where the cut off value is > 1 mm). Right ventricular infarction occurs in about 40% of patients with inferior STEMI. The right ventricular branch occurs soon after the origin of the right coronary artery. Therefore, in a patient with inferior STEMI of the left ventricle who also has right ventricular infarction, the culprit artery must be the right coronary artery and not the left circumflex artery, and the site of the lesion causing both these infarctions must be situated in the proximal part of the right coronary artery, before origin of the right ventricular branch.

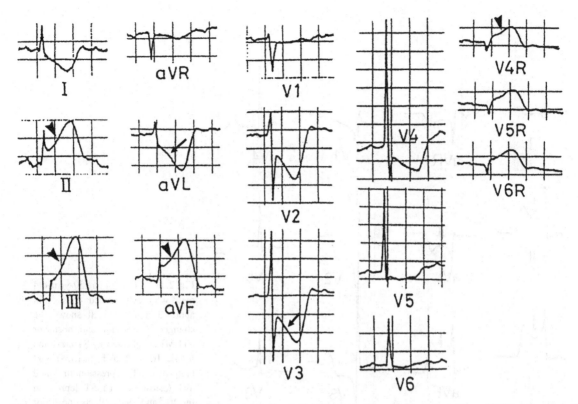

Fig. 2.9 Inferior and posterior STEMI and right ventricular infarction in a 60-year-old woman. Note: (1) ST elevation in II, III and aVF, concave upwards (arrowheads) merging with tall T waves and reciprocal ST depression in I and aVL (arrow in aVL) reflecting inferior STEMI. (2) ST depression in V₂ to V₄ (arrow in V₃) reflecting reciprocal changes of posterior STEMI. (3) ST elevation (arrowhead in V₄R) in V₄R, V₅R and V₆R reflecting acute right ventricular infarction.

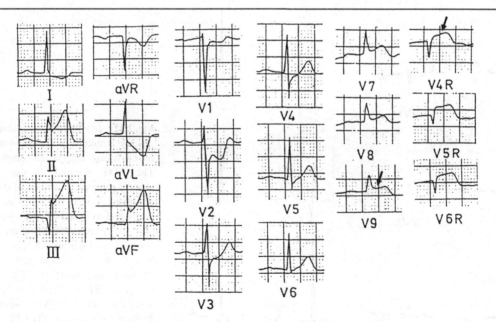

Fig. 2.10 Inferior and posterior STEMI and right ventricular infarction in a 49-year-old man. Note: (1) ST elevation in II, III and aVF (associated with pathological Q wave in III) and reciprocal ST depression in I and aVL reflecting inferior STEMI. (2) **ST elevation in V₇, V₈, V₉ (arrow in V₉)** and reciprocal ST depression in V₁ to V₃ reflecting posterior STEMI. (3) ST elevation (arrow in V₄R) in V₄R, V₅R and V₆R reflecting acute right ventricular infarction. (4) First degree AV block (PR interval = 0.28 sec).

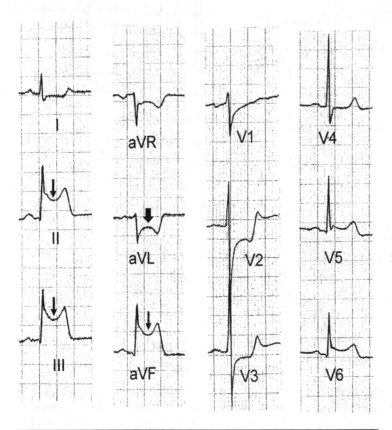

Fig. 2.11 ECG of a 50-year-old man who experienced chest pain about 3 hours ago. It shows the changes of inferior and posterior STEMI as reflected by ST elevation in II, III and aVF (arrows) and reciprocal ST depression in I and aVL (arrow in aVL). ST depression in V_2 and V_3 reflects posterior STEMI (see text in page 27).

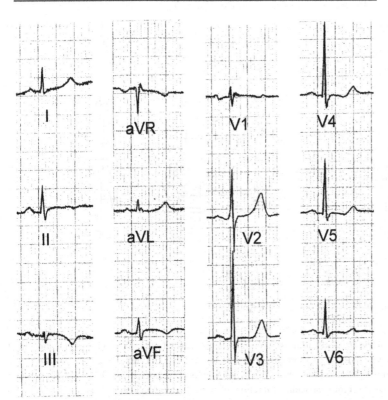

Fig. 2.12 10 minutes after sublingual glyceryl trinitrate was administered, the chest pain disappeared completely. The ECG repeated at that time showed complete resolution of the ST elevation. T wave inversion is seen in III and aVF and ST depression is seen in V_4 and V_5. Soon afterwards, coronary angiography was performed and it showed normal and patent coronary arteries (Fig. 2.13). Most likely, the ST elevation seen in Fig. 2.11 is due to coronary vasospasm – **Prinzmetal's angina**. (The ECGs in Figs. 2.11 and 2.12 are by courtesy of Clinical A/Prof Gerald Chua and Associate Professor Sin Fai Lam).

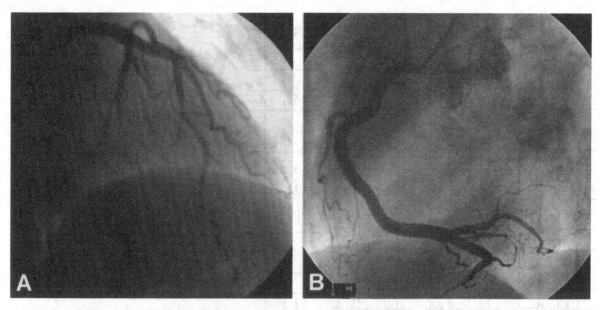

Fig. 2.13 Left and right coronary angiograms (Panels A and B respectively) in the patient whose ECGs are shown in Figs. 2.11 and 2.12. They were done after sublingual (followed by intravenous) glyceryl trinitrate was given and the chest pain had subsided. Both coronary angiograms were completely normal.

PRINZMETAL's ANGINA or CORONARY VASOSPASM

Prinzmetal's angina or variant angina is uncommon and is due to vasospasm of the coronary arteries which are either normal or are mildly or severely diseased. Such patients, unlike those with stable angina, usually experience chest pain spontaneously, especially in the early hours of the morning. The ECG recorded during an attack of chest pain will show elevated ST segments with reciprocal ST segment depression, thus resembling very closely anterior or inferior STEMI. However unlike STEMI, the ECG quickly becomes normal when the chest pain subsides when sublingual glyceryl trinitrate is administered (Figs. 2.11 and 2.12). Cardiac arrhythmias such as frequent ventricular ectopic beats, ventricular tachycardia, ventricular fibrillation and atrioventricular (AV) block may all be encountered during an attack of Prinzmetal's angina.

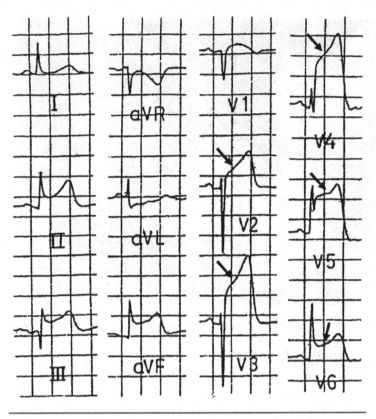

Fig. 2.14 Anterior and inferior STEMI. Note: ST elevation in V_2-V_6 (arrows) and in II, III and aVF. The sum total of the ST elevation in the 12 leads = 41 mm. Coronary angiography showed a 90% stenosis of the mid-left anterior descending artery (LAD). After successful percutaneous coronary intervention (PCI) with stenting, it was noted that the LAD was a wrap around artery. (ECGs in Figs. 2.14 and 2.15 courtesy of Professor Huay-Cheem Tan).

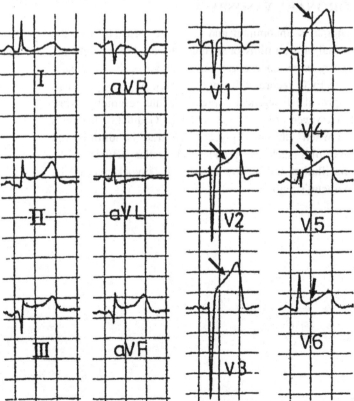

Fig. 2.15 ECG after successful PCI and stenting. The ST elevation has decreased significantly especially in V_2 to V_6 (arrows). The sum total of the ST elevation in the 12 leads = 22 mm, which is a significant reduction of 46% compared to the pre-PCI ECG (see text in page 29).

ECG in STEMI after THROMBOLYTIC THERAPY or PERCUTANEUS CORONARY INTERVENTION

A 12-lead ECG is strongly recommended to be repeated soon after the completion of thrombolytic therapy or percutaneous coronary intervention. If there is significant resolution of the ST segment elevation, it is likely that reperfusion has been achieved and prognosis is favourable (Figs. 2.14 and 2.15).

HYPERACUTE TALL T WAVES AS THE FIRST PRESENTING ECG ABNORMALITY IN STEMI

Occasionally, the first ECG change in STEMI is symmetrical, broad-based T waves, which unlike hyperkalaemia are not pointed and peaked (Fig. 2.16). ST segment elevation follows subsequently. Another different type of hyperacute tall T wave called the De Winter T wave is discussed in the Epilogue section in page 45.

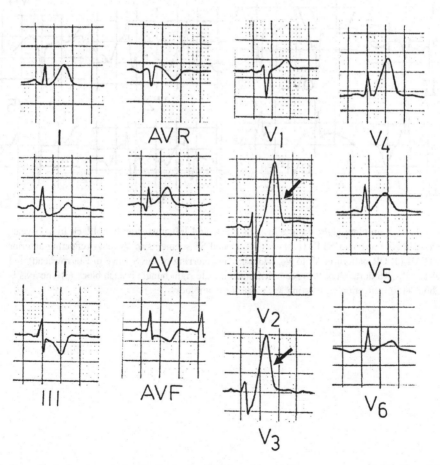

Fig. 2.16 ECG of a patient who presented with chest pain. Tall, broad based T waves are seen in V_2, V_3 and V_4 (arrows in V_2 and V_3). The T wave in V_2 = 17 mm. ST depression/T wave inversion is present in II, III, aVF and ST elevation is seen in aVR. Several hours later, a repeat ECG shows fully evolved pattern of anterior STEMI.

DIAGNOSIS of STEMI in COMPLETE RIGHT and LEFT BUNDLE BRANCH BLOCK

STEMI is easily diagnosed in patients with complete right bundle branch block. The initial r wave is obliterated resulting in a QR complex. ST segment elevation is not affected (Fig. 2.17). In contrast, the diagnosis of STEMI when complete left bundle branch block is present is complicated and difficult. Many diagnostic criteria have been proposed but none is entirely satisfactory. Perhaps the best criterion is concordant ST segment elevation (i.e. ST segment elevation in leads showing dominant R waves) which has a very high specificity, but unfortunately a low sensitivity (Fig. 2.18).

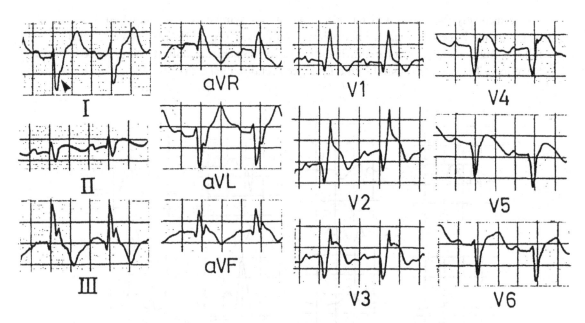

Fig. 2.17 Complete right bundle branch block and left posterior hemiblock in a 53-year-old man with **anterior STEMI**. Note: (1) Elevated ST segments in V_1 to V_4 reflecting anterior STEMI (2) QR pattern in V_1 to V_3, widening and slurring of the S wave in I (arrowhead) and aVL and QRS duration of 0.16 sec reflecting complete right bundle branch block (3) The axis is about +150° reflecting co-existing left posterior hemiblock.

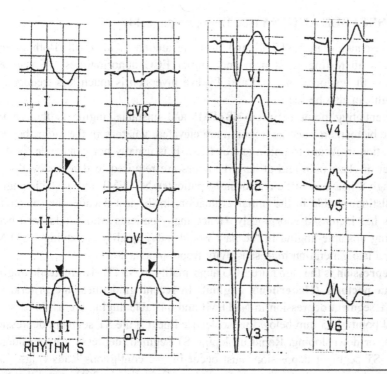

Fig. 2.18 ECG showing **complete left bundle branch block and inferior STEMI**. Note: (1) Widened M shaped QRS complex in V_6 (QRS duration = 0.16 sec) indicating complete left bundle branch block (2) Concordant ST elevation in II, III and aVF (arrowheads) and pathological Q waves in III and aVF. Reciprocal ST depression in I and aVL. These changes indicate inferior STEMI.

REINFARCTION

A frequent clinical problem is the diagnosis of reinfarction in a patient who had previously suffered a myocardial infarction and now complains of chest pain. In this situation, a comparison of a new ECG with the previous stable ECGs and cardiac biomarkers are both useful (Fig. 2.19).

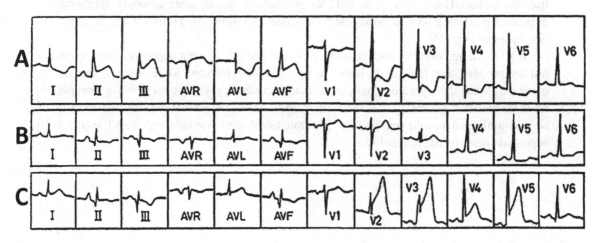

Fig. 2.19 Reinfarction. Top panel (A). ECG of a patient presenting with chest pain. It shows inferior STEMI as reflected by ST elevation in II, III and aVF and reciprocal ST depression in I and aVL. Posterior STEMI is also present as reflected by ST depression in V_2 to V_5. Middle panel (B) ECG a few months later showing resolution phase of inferior STEMI as reflected by pathological Q waves and inverted T waves in III and aVF. Bottom panel (C) Many months later, the patient experienced chest pain again. ECG now shows anterior STEMI as reflected by ST elevation in V_2 to V_5 associated with tall T waves. Evidence of resolution phase of inferior STEMI is now more prominent – the Q waves in III and aVF are wider and deeper and the T waves are deeper compared to those seen in panel B.

NSTEMI and UNSTABLE ANGINA (see Epilogue page 44)

The clinical presentation in NSTEMI and unstable angina is identical. Both groups of patients present with resting chest pain and similar ECG abnormalities. ST segment depression occurs in the majority of cases and T wave inversion is much less frequent. A combination of both can also be seen.

The key differentiating point between NSTEMI and unstable angina is that in the former, the cardiac biomarkers such as troponin are elevated, whereas in the latter they are not. Since an elevation in serum troponin and/or CK-MB is usually not detectable for 4 to 6 hours after onset of chest pain and at least 12 hours are required to detect elevation in all patients (although 8 hours is sufficient for most patients), NSTEMI and unstable angina are frequently indistinguishable in the initial evaluation. In the last decade, the sensitivity of troponin assays has increased enormously. Hence many patients who would have been diagnosed as having unstable angina in the past would today qualify as having NSTEMI when tested using a late generation high sensitivity troponin assay.

ST segment depression is the signature ECG abnormality in **NSTEMI, unstable angina and stable angina pectoris (Heberden's angina)**. In recent guidelines, the criteria for diagnosing new ST segment depression in NSTEMI and unstable angina are as follows: (1) depression of the J point ≥ 0.5 mm below the isoelectric line. (2) the ST segment depression must be horizontal or downsloping. Rapid upsloping ST segment depression is considered as benign. (3) the ST segment depression must occur in ≥ 2 contiguous leads (Figs. 2.20 and 2.21). However, the European Society of Cardiology Guideline in 2011 stated that "ST segment depression ≥ 0.05 mV (*which is equivalent to 0.5 mm*) in 2 or more contiguous leads in the appropriate context, is suggestive of NSTE-ACS (*NSTEMI and unstable angina*) and linked to prognosis. Minor 0.05 mV (*0.5 mm*) ST depression may be difficult to measure in clinical practice. More relevant is ST depression > 0.1 mV (*1 mm*) which is associated with an 11% death rate and myocardial infarction at 1 year" (italics in brackets from the author). Hamm CW et al. ESC for the management of acute coronary syndrome in patients presenting without persistent ST-segment elevation. Eur Heart J 2011; 32: 2999. (see Epilogue page 44).

In NSTEMI and unstable angina, both chest pain and ST segment depression are seen at rest and are persistent. In contrast, in angina pectoris, chest pain and ST segment depression occur only when the myocardial oxygen demand exceeds supply. This happens for example when the patient is exercising or is mentally stressed. When the patient stops exercising or if he is administered a sublingual glyceryl trinitrate tablet, the chest pain and the ST segment depression often recede gradually.

In all the above 3 situations where subendocardial myocardial ischaemia is the dominant factor, the ST segment depression is maximum in leads V_4 to V_6. In contrast, in the reciprocal ST segment depression resulting from posterior STEMI, the maximum ST segment depression is from V_1 to V_3.

Unlike ST segment elevation or Q waves, ST segment depression generally cannot localize the coronary artery that is involved. However, the deeper the ST segment depression and the more leads they occur in, the more likely the patient has severe coronary artery disease. If > 1 mm ST segment depression is found in ≥ 8 leads and if the ST segment is elevated in lead aVR and/or lead V_1, it is very likely that the patient has left main or triple vessel disease and requires urgent coronary angiography (Fig. 2.21).

Apart from myocardial ischaemia, the non-ischaemic causes of ST segment depression include reciprocal ST segment depression arising from STEMI, left and right ventricular hypertrophy with strain pattern, secondary ST-T wave changes in left bundle branch block, and acute pulmonary embolism.

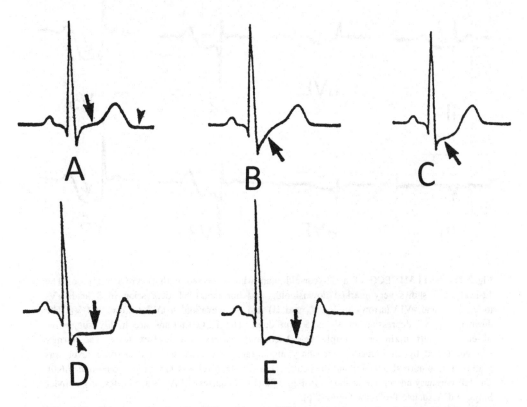

Fig. 2.20 Diagram showing the different types of **ST segment depression** indicated by arrows (A) ST segment with no deflection (arrowhead indicates isoelectric line) (B) Rapid upsloping ST segment depression (C) Slow upsloping ST segment depression (D) Horizontal ST segment depression (arrowhead shows J point/ST segment depression (E) Downsloping ST segment depression **(see page 32, 33 and Epilogue page 44)**.

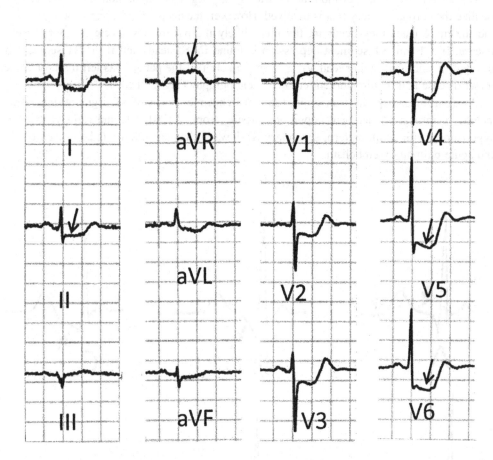

Fig. 2.21 NSTEMI. ECG of a 62-year-old man who presented with severe chest pain. The 12-lead ECG shows very marked downsloping and horizontal ST depression in 8 leads (V_2 to V_6, I, II and aVL) (arrows in V_5, V_6 and II) and ST elevation in aVR (arrow) and V_1. The downsloping ST depression in V_5 is 5 mm deep. The ECG findings are highly suggestive of either a **left main** or a **triple vessel** coronary artery disease (see text). The former was confirmed by an immediate coronary angiogram. The peak serum troponin l level was > 80 ug/L (top normal = 0.039) and the peak serum CKMB level was 175 ug/L (top normal = 6.0). The left coronary angiogram is shown in Fig. 2.22 (ECG courtesy of Assistant Professor Devinder Singh and Associate Professor James Yip).

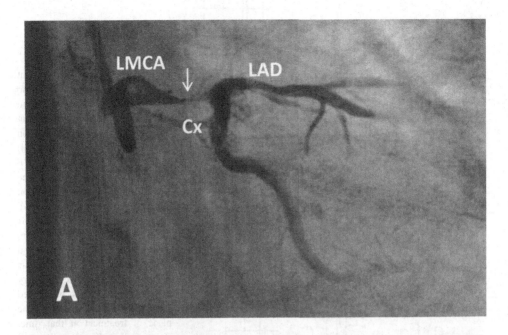

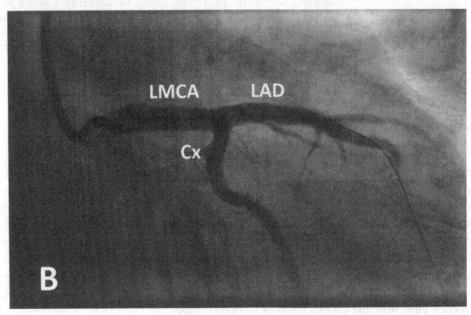

Fig. 2.22 Top panel (A) Left coronary angiogram in the right anterior oblique view of the patient whose ECG is shown in Fig. 2.21. There is a diffuse 99% subocclusive stenosis in the distal left main coronary artery (LMCA) indicated by a down pointing arrow. The left anterior descending artery (LAD) shows a 70% stenosis. The left circumflex artery (Cx) is normal. The mid-right coronary artery is totally occluded (not shown). Bottom panel (B) Shows the left coronary angiogram after successful PCI and stenting of the LMCA and the LAD. Both arteries are now completely patent. Three days later, PCI and stenting of the total occlusion of the mid-right coronary artery was successfully achieved. The patient's hospital stay and recovery was uneventful. (Coronary angiograms courtesy of Assistant Professor Poay-Huan Loh).

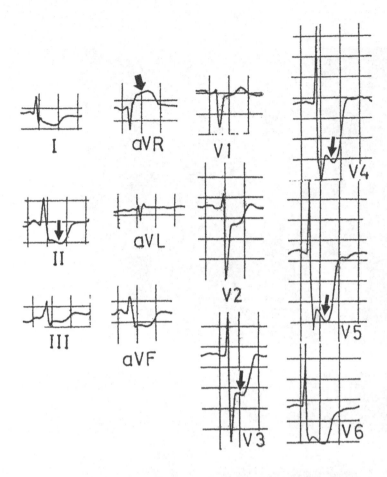

Fig. 2.23 NSTEMI. The patient was a 54-year-old man who presented with severe chest pain and cardiogenic shock. Note that there is very deep ST depression (downsloping and horizontal) in V_2 to V_6, I, II, III and aVF (arrows in V_3 to V_5 and II). The deepest ST segment depression (14 mm) is seen in V_5 (arrow). There is also ST elevation in aVR (arrow). The cardiac biomarkers were all markedly elevated and the patient was diagnosed as having severe NSTEMI. Coronary angiography was not performed because it was not available in the place of treatment at that time. But the clinical presentation and ECG strongly suggested that the patient was suffering from either left main or triple coronary artery disease. Despite optimal medical treatment, the patient died.

INVERTED T WAVE AND GIANT T WAVE INVERSION (see page 66)

In acute myocardial ischaemia, an inverted T wave is defined as a ≥ 1 mm T wave inversion in a lead where the R wave is dominant. It should occur in ≥ 2 contiguous leads. Apart from ischaemic heart disease (NSTEMI, unstable angina and stable angina), the other causes of mildly inverted T waves are innumerable as discussed in page 66. If the T wave is inverted ≥ 10 mm in ≥ 2 contiguous leads, it is described as giant T wave inversion. Here, the causes are more limited. In patients with any of the causes of giant T wave inversion listed below, the amplitude of the T wave inversion frequently may not be as deep as ≥ 10 mm, but may be around 5 mm. There are many other causes of moderate T wave inversion, including acute myocarditis, stage 3 resolving phase of acute pericarditis, acute pulmonary embolism and various types of cardiomyopathy.

Causes of Giant T Wave Inversion

(1) NSTEMI (symmetrical)
(2) Fully evolved or resolved phases of STEMI (symmetrical)
(3) Left/right ventricular hypertrophy with strain pattern (asymmetrical)
(4) Hypertrophic cardiomyopathy (especially apical variety)
(5) Takotsubo cardiomyopathy
(6) Intracranial haemorrhage (especially subarachnoid haemorrhage [symmetrical])

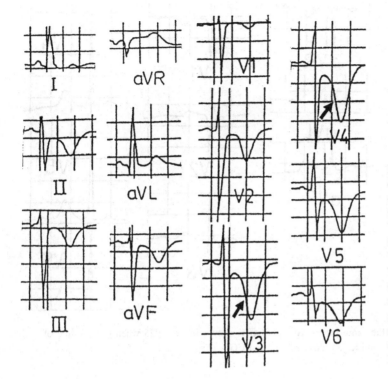

Fig. 2.24 NSTEMI. A 65-year-old woman presented with severe chest pain. ECG shows marked ST segment depression in V_2 to V_6 and symmetrical giant T wave inversion in V_3 to V_5 (arrows in V_3 and V_4) and lesser degree of T wave inversion in other leads. Coronary angiography showed severe stenosis of the proximal left anterior descending artery. The cardiac biomarkers were elevated and she was diagnosed as having NSTEMI.

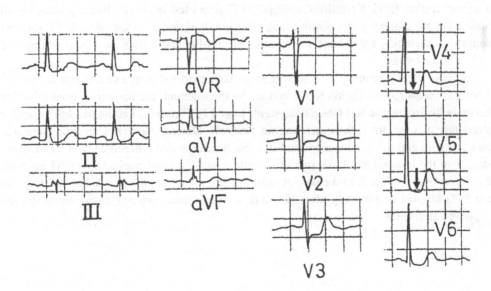

Fig. 2.25 Unstable angina. ECG of a 60-year-old man with chest pain at rest. ECG shows marked ST depression from V_3 to V_6 (arrows in V_4 and V_5). The cardiac biomarkers were not elevated. Subsequent coronary angiography showed 90% stenosis of the mid left anterior descending artery.

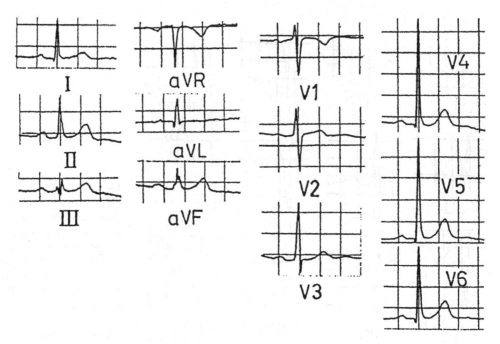

Fig. 2.26 ECG of the same patient whose ECG is shown in Fig. 2.25 when he was free of chest pain. No abnormalities are detected in this ECG.

EXERCISE ECG STRESS TEST

In patients who are suspected of suffering from coronary artery disease but who have a normal resting ECG, a treadmill exercise ECG stress test using the Bruce protocol is an option. For the diagnosis of a positive test, a ≥ 1 mm horizontal or downsloping ST segment depression persisting for at least 0.08 second (80 milliseconds) after the J point is required in 1 or more leads.

Because the TP segment is absent in sinus tachycardia during exercise stress test, the J point is measured in relation to the end of the PR segment, the horizontal level of which becomes the isoelectric line **(see ST segment, page 12)**. Figure 2.27 is the treadmill exercise stress test in a patient with **severe angina pectoris**. During the resting period, there was no chest pain and the ECG was normal (the machine recorded a modified lead V_5). During stage 1 of the test and at a heart rate of 107/min, chest pain and marked 6 mm ST segment depression were induced. In the post-exercise period, the chest pain receded completely and the ECG became normal only after 12 minutes. Subsequent coronary angiography showed triple vessel disease.

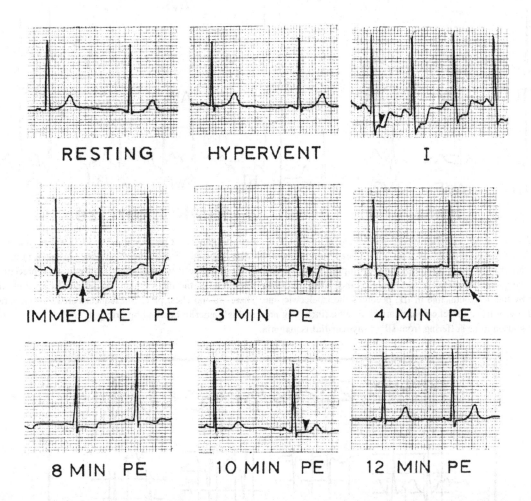

RESTING HYPERVENT I

IMMEDIATE PE 3 MIN PE 4 MIN PE

8 MIN PE 10 MIN PE 12 MIN PE

Fig. 2.27 Treadmill exercise stress testing in a 52-year-old man with severe angina pectoris. The patient experienced chest pain during Stage 1 of the Bruce exercise stress test protocol and the test was stopped. ECG was recorded using a modified V_5 lead. The resting ECG and that recorded after hyperventilation (HYPERVENT) were both normal. There was no chest pain then. There was 6 mm ST segment depression (arrowhead) accompanied by chest pain in Stage 1. The following changes were seen in the post-exercise (PE) period. (1) Horizontal ST segment depression (arrowhead) and U wave inversion (arrow) in the immediate phase. (2) Downsloping ST segment depression (arrowhead) at 3 minutes. (3) Deeply inverted T wave (arrow) at 4 minutes. (4) Normalization of the ST segment (arrowhead) at 10 minutes. (5) Normal ECG and chest pain receded completely at 12 minutes. **See text in page 38**.

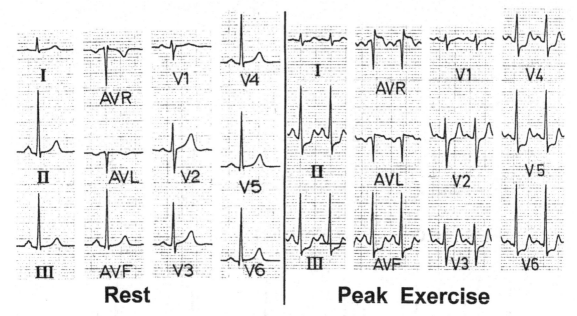

Fig. 2.28 Treadmill exercise stress test of an asymptomatic 63-year-old woman. (Left hand panel) The ECG was normal at rest. (Right hand panel) At peak exercise, with a heart rate of about 160/min, marked ST segment depression was seen in multiple leads – **horizontal** in V₅ & V₆ and **slow upsloping** in II, III & aVF. Because the P wave is superimposed on the preceding T wave during sinus tachycardia, the J point is measured in relation to the end of the PR segment, the horizontal level of which (shown by the horizontal line in III) becomes the isoelectric line. There was no chest pain. Subsequent coronary angiography showed severe triple vessel coronary artery disease (including proximal left anterior descending artery disease). The patient was thus diagnosed to be suffering from **silent myocardial ischaemia**.

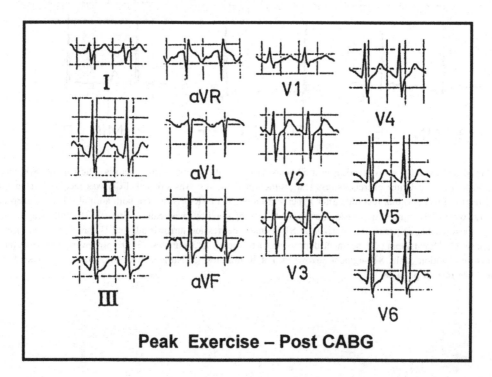

Fig. 2.29 ECG at peak exercise of the same patient whose ECG is shown in Fig. 2.28, after coronary artery bypass surgery (CABG). At a heart rate of about 150/min, the ECG was normal, indicating an absence of myocardial ischaemia as a result of successful myocardial revascularization.

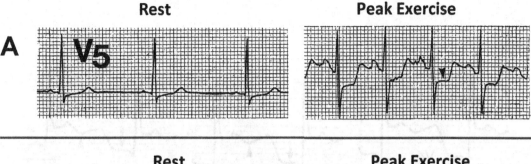

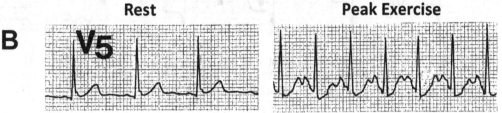

Fig. 2.30   Angina pectoris. Treadmill exercise stress test in a patient with angina pectoris and left main coronary artery disease. The upper panel (A) was recorded before coronary artery bypass surgery was done. At peak exercise with a heart rate of about 108/min, the patient experienced chest pain and a 5 mm horizontal ST depression in V_5 (arrowhead) was seen. Both these findings indicate severe angina pectoris. The bottom panel (B) was recorded after successful coronary artery bypass surgery. At peak exercise, and a heart rate of about 150/min, there was no chest pain and the ECG was normal indicating successful myocardial revascularization.

U WAVE INVERSION

In recent years, the importance of U wave inversion as a specific ECG marker of heart disease such as myocardial ischaemia, hypertensive and myocardial disease has been re-emphasized (Figs. 2.31 to 2.33). In ischaemic heart disease, U wave inversion is usually associated with ST segment depression (Fig. 2.32). However, it may rarely be the sole abnormality. A previous study reported that exercise induced inversion of the praecordial U waves was correlated with severe stenosis of the left anterior descending artery.

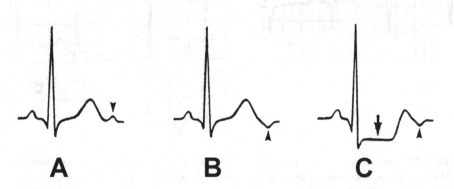

Fig. 2.31   Diagram showing: (A) Normal upright U wave (arrowhead). (B) Isolated U wave inversion (arrowhead). (C) U wave inversion (arrowhead) associated with ST segment depression (arrow).

41

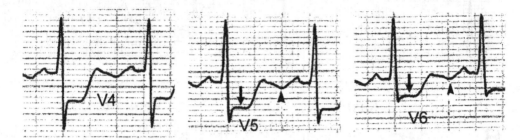

Fig. 2.32 NSTEMI. ECG of a patient with NSTEMI. Marked horizontal/downsloping ST segment is seen in multiple leads in the 12-lead ECG. In leads V_4, V_5 and V_6, in addition to the ST segment depression (arrows in V_5 and V_6), **inverted U waves** (arrowheads in V_5 and V_6) are seen.

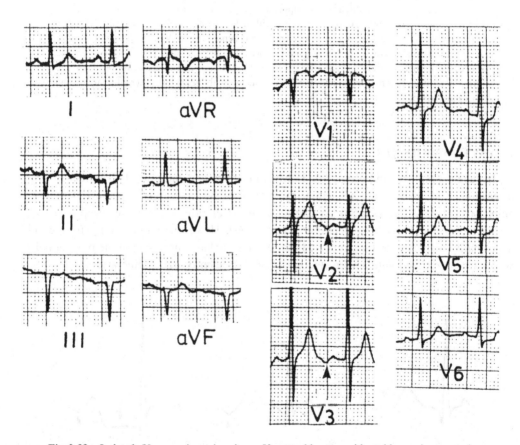

Fig. 2.33 Isolated U wave inversion in a 50-year-old man with stable angina pectoris. U wave inversion, without ST segment depression, is seen in V_2 and V_3 (arrowheads). The axis is about $-50°$ reflecting left anterior hemiblock. Coronary angiography showed a 99% narrowing of the proximal left anterior descending artery.

VENTRICULAR ECTOPIC BEATS

The polarity of the T wave in ventricular ectopic beats is opposite to that of the QRS complex. It is therefore inverted when the ventricular complex shows a predominant R wave, and upright when it shows a predominant S wave. The ST segment blends smoothly and imperceptibly with the T wave whose 2 limbs are asymmetrical. The following deviations in the morphology of the ventricular ectopic beat suggest underlying ischaemic or myocardial disease: (1) **Deep and symmetrically inverted T wave** (Fig. 2.34) (2) T wave polarity identical to that of the qRS complex (3) presence of a q wave in a ventricular ectopic beat with a predominant R or Rs complex (Fig. 2.35).

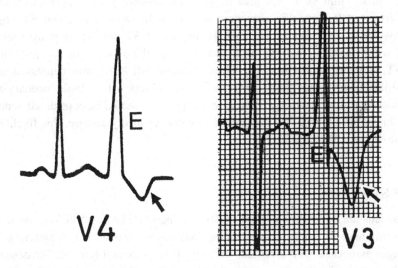

Fig. 2.34 The left hand panel shows a ventricular ectopic beat (E) in a normal individual. The T wave is not deep and the 2 limbs are asymmetrical. The right hand panel shows a ventricular ectopic beat (E) in a patient with previous NSTEMI. The T wave of the ventricular ectopic beat is deep and symmetrical (arrow).

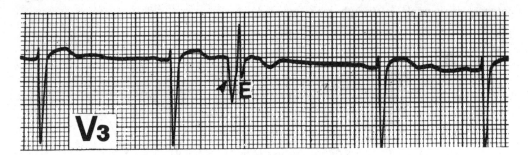

Fig. 2.35 ECG of a patient who had previously suffered a transmural myocardial infarction. Although the rS complex of the sinus beat is essentially normal except for a slightly coved ST segment, the predominant R wave ventricular ectopic beat (E) shows a very wide and deep pathological Q wave (arrowhead) indicating an old, transmural myocardial infarction.

EPILOGUE

Criteria for the ECG diagnosis of both left main coronary artery occlusion and proximal versus mid/distal left anterior descending artery occlusion in anterior STEMI and right coronary artery versus left circumflex artery occlusion in inferior STEMI have all been reported. However, they are beyond the scope of this book.

In recent guidelines, the criteria for diagnosing new ST segment depression in NSTEMI and unstable angina is ≥ 0.5 mm. However, the European Society of Cardiology Guideline (2011) has suggested an alternative cutoff value of > 1 mm, because it may be difficult to measure minor 0.5 mm ST segment depression in clinical practice. The advantages and disadvantages of 0.5 mm vs 1 mm also depends on sensitivity and specificity; 0.5 mm is more sensitive but less specific compared to 1 mm. In **rapid upsloping ST segment depression** (which is regarded as normal) the depressed ST segment rapidly returns to the baseline within 0.08 second (80 milliseconds) after the J point. In contrast, in **slow upsloping ST segment depression**, the ST segment is still ≥ 1.5 mm depressed at 0.08 second (80 milliseconds) after the J point. In patient subsets with a high coronary artery disease prevalence, a slow upsloping ST segment depression should be considered abnormal. However, in individuals with a low prevalence of coronary artery disease, this likelihood is less certain **(See page 32 and 33)**.

WELLENS SYNDROME

Most clinicians are quite clear in their understanding of STEMI, NSTEMI, and unstable angina, but some have difficulty understanding Wellens Syndrome. It is a pattern of ECG T wave changes associated with a critical stenosis of the proximal left anterior descending artery and is a pre-infarction stage of unstable angina. However, when the patient is seen, the chest pain has receded and the cardiac enzymes are either normal or minimally elevated. The ECG shows mainly deep symmetrical T wave inversion in leads V_1 to V_4 (less often in leads V_5 and V_6). Less frequently biphasic T waves with the ST segment being either isoelectric or minimally elevated are seen (Fig. 2.36). There is a very high risk for extensive anterior myocardial infarction within the next 2-3 weeks. Therefore, early coronary angiography is strongly recommended.

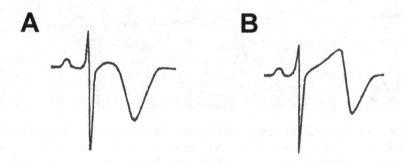

Fig. 2.36 Wellens Syndrome (A) Deeply inverted and symmetrical T wave. (B) Biphasic T wave. The preceding ST segment is not elevated.

"De WINTER" T WAVE

The De Winter ECG pattern was first described in 2008 (de Winter RJ, Verouden NJ, Wellens HJ, Wilde AA. A new ECG sign of proximal LAD occlusion. N Engl J Med 2008; 359: 2071). This pattern signifies acute occlusion of the proximal left anterior descending artery.

The ECG begins with a > 1 mm upsloping ST segment depression at the J point in leads V_1 to V_6 continuing into tall, upright symmetrical T waves. In most cases, 0.5-1 mm ST segment elevation is seen in lead aVR. Unlike the hyperacute broad T waves described earlier in page 29 (Fig. 2.16) where ST segment elevation follows subsequently, De Winter T waves are generally persistent right up to the moment of percutaneous coronary intervention. Urgent coronary angiogram is usually performed in patients showing de Winter T waves.

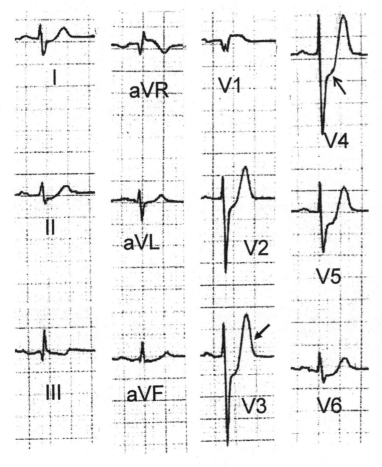

Fig. 2.37 De Winter T wave. The 12-lead ECG was recorded in a 57-year-old man 2 hours after the onset of chest pain. Prominent upsloping ST segment depression (up pointing arrow in V_4) is seen in V_2 to V_5, continuing upwards into tall symmetrical T waves (down pointing arrow in V_3). In V_4, 5 mm ST depression is seen, and in V_3, the T wave is 10 mm tall. 2 mm ST elevation is seen in aVR. Coronary angiography showed triple vessel coronary artery disease with 90% stenosis of both the proximal left anterior descending artery and the left circumflex artery, and 70% stenosis of the right coronary artery. Successful PCI and stenting of the left anterior descending and the left circumflex arteries were performed (ECG courtesy of Associate Professor Ronald Chi-Hang Lee and Assistant Professor Edgar Tay).

CHAPTER 3

MISCELLANEOUS CONDITIONS

NORMAL MALE PATTERN

In a study of 529 normal males, it was found that ≥ 1 mm ST elevation in one or more of the leads V_1 to V_4 was seen in 91% of those who were between 17-24 years. This prevalence of ST elevation however decreased to 14% in those who were 76 years and older (Surawicz B et al. J Am Coll Cardiol 2002; 40: 1870). This very high prevalence of ST elevation (especially in leads V_2 and V_3) in young normal males (Fig. 3.1) has been termed "normal male pattern" (Wang K. Atlas of Electrocardiography, page 223. Jaypee Brothers Medical Publishers (P) Ltd, 2013). In contrast, the prevalence of ≥ 1 mm ST elevation in one or more of the leads V_1 to V_4 is about 10-20% in females and remains mostly constant throughout the different age groups.

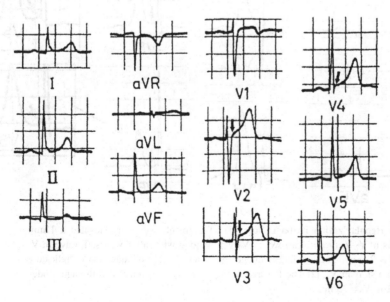

Fig. 3.1 12-lead ECG in a normal young man. Note ST elevation in V_2 to V_4 (arrows) reflecting the normal male pattern.

EARLY REPOLARIZATION PATTERN

The Early Repolarization Pattern has been recognized for the past few decades. The J point is elevated ≥ 1 mm in ≥ 2 contiguous leads in leads V_3 to V_6. Less commonly, this pattern can also been seen in the limb leads. At the elevated J point, there is frequently either a notch or a slurr, followed by a concave elevation of the ST segment which slopes upwards, merging with a tall T wave. In addition, the left praecordial R waves are also usually tall (Fig. 3.2). This pattern is seen in about 5% of the general population and is common in young men and athletes.

For decades, this pattern has been regarded as totally benign. However, in the past few years, there has been a controversy whether this pattern carries a very small risk of ventricular fibrillation. Most likely, the reported cases of Early Repolarization Pattern and ventricular fibrillation belong to a different entity. This is because many of these patients do not show ST elevation, but instead exhibit a horizontal or downsloping ST segment.

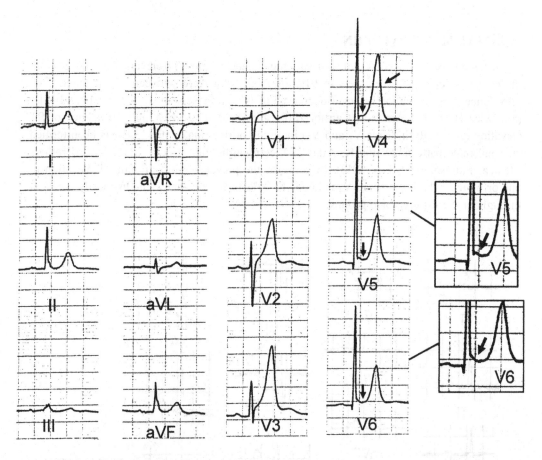

Fig. 3.2 Early Repolarization Pattern. Note: (1) ST segments which are elevated ≥ 1 mm concave upwards in V_2-V_6 (vertical arrows in V_4-V_6) merging with tall T waves. T wave in V_4 (oblique arrow) is 21 mm. In the enlarged images of V_5 and V_6, the oblique arrows indicate a notch in V_5 and a slurr in V_6. (2) The R waves in V_4 to V_6 are prominent and the amplitudes are increased. R in V_5 = 35 mm.

ACUTE PERICARDITIS

In acute pericarditis, there is widespread elevation of the ST segments (concave upwards). Frequently, ST segment depression is present only in lead aVR and the ST segment is isoelectric in lead aVL (Fig. 3.3). This is because in acute pericarditis, the ST segment vector in the frontal plane is directed towards lead II, resulting in maximum ST segment elevation in this lead, and reciprocal ST segment depression in lead aVR. In contrast, in inferior STEMI, the maximum ST segment elevation is usually between leads III and aVF.

Maximal elevation of the ST segment in lead II, with lesser degrees of ST elevation in the other limb leads, together with widespread ST segment elevation in the praecordial leads, also help to distinguish acute pericarditis from STEMI and the early repolarization pattern. A further point of distinction between acute pericarditis and the early repolarization pattern is that the height of the T waves in the former is normal, whereas it is considerably increased in the latter. As a result of this, the ST/T ratio (i.e. the height of ST segment elevation divided by the amplitude of the T wave) in lead V_6 and other left praecordial leads is > 0.25 in acute pericarditis, and < 0.25 in the early repolarization pattern. Lastly, in acute pericarditis, there is depression of the PR segment in many leads but frequently maximal in lead II. The QRS voltages in patients with acute pericarditis, but without pericardial effusion, are normal.

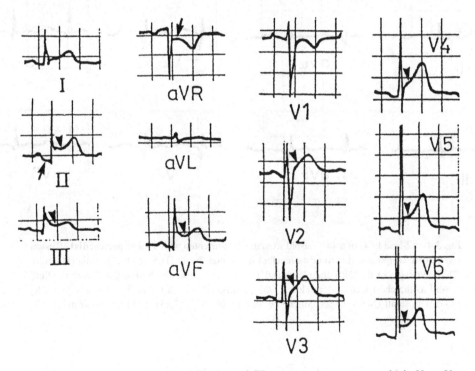

Fig. 3.3 Acute pericarditis. Note: (1) Elevated ST segments (concave upwards) in V_2 to V_6, II, III and aVF (arrowheads). The ST segment elevation in the limb leads is maximal in II. (2) ST segment depression in aVR (arrow). (3) Depressed PR segment in II (arrow). (4) Normal QRS and T wave voltages.

PERICARDIAL EFFUSION

In large pericardial effusions, the voltages of the QRS complexes, the P waves and the T waves are all considerably diminished in the limb and praecordial leads (Fig. 3.4). Occasionally, electrical **QRS alternans** (i.e. alternation of the height or axis of the QRS complexes) is present, especially in very large, pericardial effusions with cardiac tamponade (Fig. 3.6).

Currently, echocardiography has enabled the diagnosis of pericardial effusion to be confirmed easily and accurately. Figure 3.5 is the two-dimensional echocardiogram of a patient demonstrating a large pericardial effusion and cardiac tamponade.

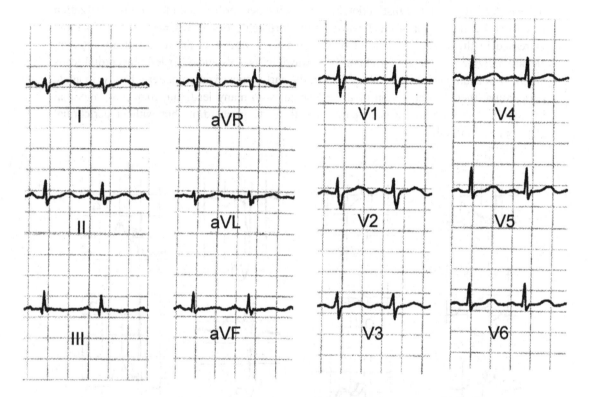

Fig. 3.4 12-lead ECG of a 48-year-old woman who presented with a **large pericardial effusion** and cardiac tamponade due to acute myeloid leukaemia. Note: (1) Sinus tachycardia (116/min). (2) The voltages of the QRS complexes and T waves are markedly diminished in both the limb as well as the chest leads. (Reproduced with permission. Low TT, Tan VS, Teo SG, Poh KK. ECGs with small QRS voltages. Singapore Med J. 2012 May; 53(5): 299 [with adaptation]).

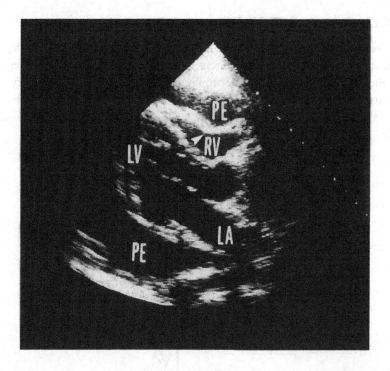

Fig. 3.5 Two-dimensional **echocardiogram** of a patient with a large pericardial effusion (PE). The frame was recorded in the parasternal long-axis view. Arrowhead indicates diastolic collapse of the right ventricle (RV) reflecting cardiac tamponade (LA = left atrium, LV = left ventricle).

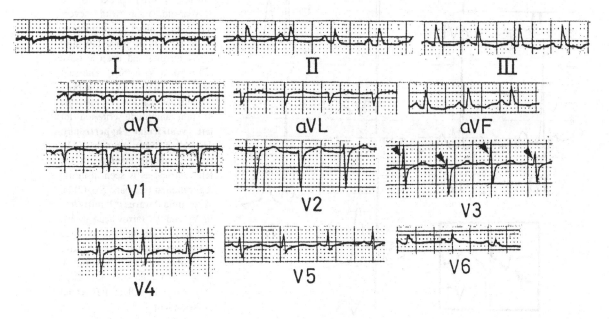

Fig. 3.6 **QRS alternans** in a patient with a very large pericardial effusion. Note: (1) Low voltages of the P, QRS and T wave complexes in both the limb as well as the praecordial leads. (2) QRS alternans which is best seen in V_1 and V_3 (arrowheads).

VENTRICULAR HYPERTROPHY (see page 55)

In **left ventricular hypertrophy**, tall R waves are seen in leads V_5 and V_6 and deep S waves in leads V_1 and V_2. Many different QRS amplitude criteria have been proposed for the diagnosis of left ventricular hypertrophy but none is entirely satisfactory. The most commonly used criterion (Sokolow–Lyon) states that $SV_1 + RV_5/RV_6$ (whichever is the taller) is > 35 mm (Fig. 3.7). This criterion has a specificity of > 90%, but a low sensitivity.

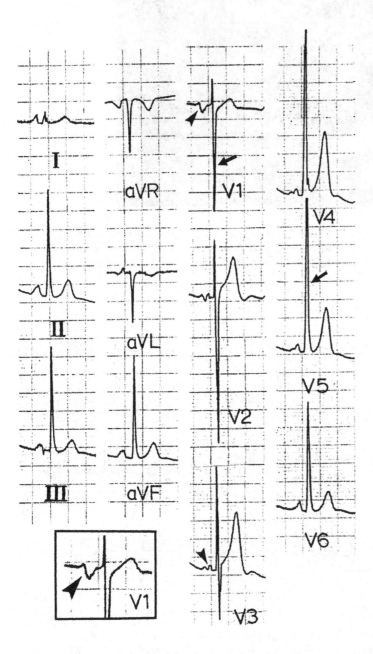

Fig. 3.7 12-lead ECG of a 36-year-old man with severe rheumatic mitral regurgitation. Note: (1) Tall R wave (40 mm) in V_5 (arrow) and deep S wave (30 mm) in V_1 (arrow). The sum of SV_1 (30 mm) + RV_5 (40 mm) = 70 mm, which far exceeds the 35 mm amplitude criterion for **left ventricular hypertrophy**. The tall T waves seen in V_3-V_5 suggest volume overload of the left ventricle as is seen in mitral regurgitation (see page 55). (2) (a) Wide, bifid P waves (**"P mitrale"**) in V_2 and V_3 (arrowhead in V_3) and (b) Wide and deep (area more than 1 small box) negative deflection of the biphasic P wave in V_1 (arrowhead). Both 2(a) and 2(b) reflect **left atrial enlargement**.

In severe left ventricular hypertrophy, ST segment depression and T wave inversion accompany tall R waves in leads V_5 and V_6 – the so-called **"left ventricular hypertrophy with strain"** pattern. Unlike in ischaemic heart disease where the T wave inversion is symmetrical, T wave inversion in left ventricular hypertrophy is usually asymmetrical, with a distal limb which is steeper than the proximal limb (Fig. 3.8). In addition, ST segment elevation is frequently seen in leads V_1 and V_2 in severe left ventricular hypertrophy and this often simulates anterior STEMI (Figs. 3.8 and 3.16).

The important causes of left ventricular hypertrophy are hypertension, valvular heart disease such as aortic stenosis, aortic regurgitation and mitral regurgitation, and hypertropic and dilated cardiomyopathy.

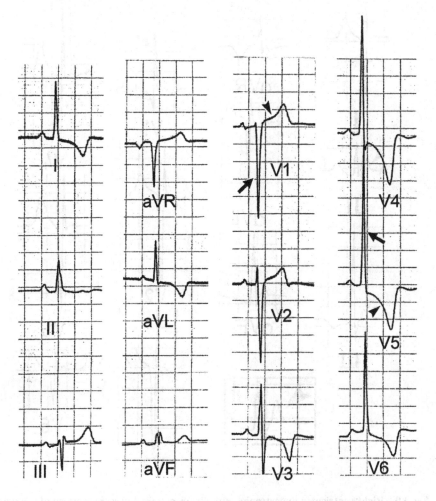

Fig. 3.8 Left ventricular hypertrophy with strain pattern (pressure overload of the left ventricle [see page 55]) in a 71-year-old man with severe uncontrolled hypertension of around 230/125 mmHg. The left ventricular hypertrophy was confirmed by two-dimensional echocardiography. Note: (1) Tall R wave (40 mm) in V_5 (arrow) (2) Deep S wave (27 mm) in V_1 (arrow) (3) SV_1 (27 mm) + RV_5 (40 mm) = 67 mm which far exceeds the amplitude criterion of 35 mm for left ventricular hypertrophy (4) ST depression and deeply inverted and asymmetrical T waves in V_4 to V_6 (arrowhead in V_5) reflecting the strain pattern (5) ST elevation which is commonly present in the right praecordial leads in severe left ventricular hypertrophy is seen in V_1 (arrowhead) and V_2 in this patient.

In **right ventricular hypertrophy**, tall R waves are seen in the right praecordial leads and deep S waves in the left praecordial leads. In lead V_1, the amplitude of the R wave is greater than that of the S wave and the R/S ratio is > 1. As in left ventricular hypertrophy, ST segment depression and T wave inversion may accompany the tall R waves if the right ventricular hypertrophy is severe (Figs. 3.9 and 3.10). Nearly always, there is also right axis deviation. The important causes of right ventricular hypertrophy are (1) pulmonary arterial hypertension which may be idiopathic, secondary to severe mitral stenosis or intracardiac shunts (2) congenital heart disease such as severe pulmonary valve stenosis and tetralogy of Fallot.

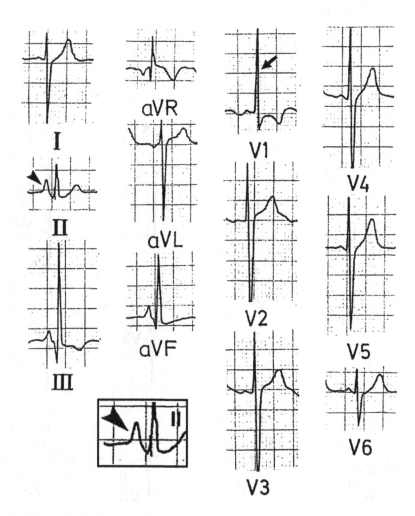

Fig. 3.9 Right ventricular hypertrophy with strain pattern (pressure overload of the right ventricle [see page 55]) and **right atrial enlargement**. Note: (1) Very tall R wave [21 mm] in V_1 (arrow). R/S ratio in V_1 = 5 (2) Right axis deviation of about +140° (3) ST depression and asymmetric T wave inversion in V_1 (4) Deep S wave in V_6 (8 mm). All these ECG abnormalities reflect right ventricular hypertrophy with strain pattern (5) Tall and peaked P wave in II [3.5 mm] (arrowhead) reflecting **right atrial enlargment ("P pulmonale")**.

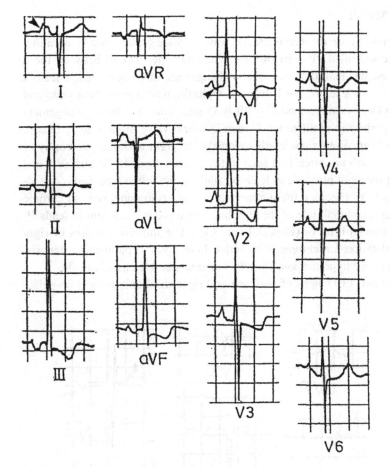

Fig. 3.10 Severe mitral stenosis with pulmonary hypertension in a 50-year-old woman. Note: (1) Left atrial enlargement as reflected by (a) a wide (0.12 sec) and bifid P wave ("P mitrale") in I (arrowhead) and aVL (b) Wide and deep negative deflection of the biphasic P wave in V_1 (arrowhead) (2) Severe right ventricular hypertrophy with strain pattern as reflected by (a) a very tall R wave in V_1 (18 mm) associated with ST segment depression and T wave inversion (b) a right axis deviation of about +120°. An ECG showing the combination of "P mitrale" and right ventricular hypertrophy is nearly always due to severe mitral stenosis with secondary pulmonary hypertension.

In 1952, Cabrera and Monroy introduced the overload concept for the ECG patterns of left and right ventricular hypertrophy (Cabrera CE, Monroy JR. Am Heart J 1952; 43: 661). Systolic overload of the left ventricle occurs when it has to pump against an increased resistance in systole, as in systemic hypertension and aortic stenosis. The ECG manifestation of **left ventricular systolic overload (similar to pressure overload)** in severe hypertension and severe aortic stenosis is reflected as the left ventricular hypertrophy with strain pattern (Fig. 3.8). Diastolic overload of the left ventricle occurs when it is overfilled in diastole, as in mitral regurgitation. The ECG manifestation of **left ventricular diastolic overload (similar to volume overload)** in severe mitral regurgitation and severe aortic regurgitation is reflected as tall R waves, deep but narrow q waves, elevated ST segments and tall T waves in the left praecordial leads (Fig. 3.7). Systolic/pressure and diastolic/volume right ventricular overload ECG patterns have also been described. The ECG manifestation of **right ventricular systolic/ pressure overload** in severe pulmonary hypertension (Fig. 3.10) and severe pulmonary valve stenosis is reflected as the right ventricular hypertrophy with strain pattern. In contrast, the ECG manifestation of **right ventricular diastolic/volume overload** in a large atrial septal defect ostium secundum (Fig. 7.4) is reflected as a right bundle branch block pattern (usually incomplete). Although the concept of pressure and volume overload had been popular, currently, it's clinical application has been found to be limited especially in patients with advanced cardiac disease, with severe dilatation and hypertrophy.

In **bi-ventricular hypertrophy,** various ECG patterns may be encountered, one of which is the presence of right axis deviation despite ECG evidence of left ventricular hypertrophy.

ATRIAL ENLARGEMENT

In **left atrial hypertrophy or dilatation**, the P wave is wide (≥ 0.12 sec in duration) and bifid in shape – the so-called **"P mitrale"** pattern. The time interval between the 2 peaks of the P wave is greater than 0.04 sec. These changes are often best seen in leads I and II and leads V_4 to V_6. In lead V_1, the P wave is biphasic, with a prominent wide and deep negative deflection (area of more than 1 small box) suggesting left atrial enlargement (Fig. 3.7). Left atrial hypertrophy or dilatation is seen in mitral valve disease, hypertensive heart disease, ischaemic heart disease and cardiomyopathy. In **right atrial hypertrophy** or **dilatation**, the P waves, which are often best seen in the inferior leads II, III and aVF, and to a lesser extent also in the right praecordial leads V_1 and V_2, are tall and peaked – the so-called **"P pulmonale"** pattern (because these abnormalities are commonly seen in chronic obstructive lung disease). The amplitude of the P pulmonale wave is ≥ 2.5 mm in leads II, III and AVF and ≥ 1.5 mm in lead V_1 (Figs. 3.9 and 3.13). The important causes of right atrial hypertrophy or dilatation are chronic obstructive lung disease, pulmonary stenosis, tetralogy of Fallot, pulmonary hypertension, Ebstein's anomaly and tricuspid atresia.

In **bi-atrial enlargement**, ECG signs of both left and right atrial enlargement co-exist.

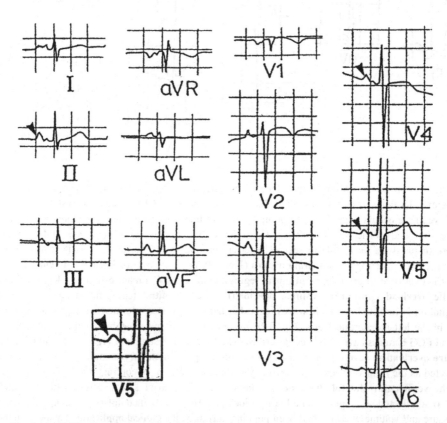

Fig. 3.11 ECG of a 34-year-old man with severe mitral stenosis and **bi-atrial enlargement** confirmed by two-dimensional echocardiography. Note (1) wide (0.12 sec) and bifid P waves in I, II, V_4 to V_6 (arrowheads in II, V_4 and V_5) indicating **"P mitrale"**, which is a reflection of left atrial enlargement. (2) In lead II, the first peak of the bifid P wave is prominent and is taller than the second peak indicating co-existence of right atrial enlargement with the left atrial enlargement.

ACUTE PULMONARY EMBOLISM

Compared to newer diagnostic modalities e.g. computed tomography pulmonary angiogram, the 12-lead ECG is not as sensitive or specific in the diagnosis of acute pulmonary embolism. Nevertheless, if the clinical evaluation is suggestive of the condition, if a previous ECG is normal and if the patient does not have preexisting cardiac or pulmonary disease, the presence of 2 or 3 of the ECG abnormalities listed below, especially abnormality 1, 2 or 3 in combination with sinus tachycardia requires the exclusion of acute pulmonary embolism.

1. S_1, Q_3, T_3 pattern (i.e. S wave in lead I, Q wave and inverted T wave in lead III)
2. Right bundle branch block
3. T wave inversion, ST segment depression or elevation in leads V_1 to V_4 and ST segment elevation in inferior leads
4. Right axis deviation
5. Clockwise rotation of the heart round its longitudinal axis, resulting in rS complexes in leads V_1 to V_5 or V_6 6. "P pulmonale"   7. Sinus tachycardia.

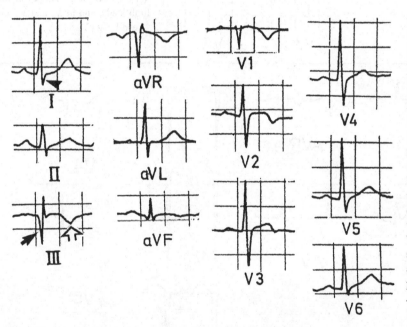

Fig. 3.12 12-lead ECG of a 30-year-old man with a proven large **pulmonary embolism**, occurring after an orthopaedic operation. Note: (1) S_1, Q_3, T_3 pattern – arrowhead in I indicates S_1, closed and open arrows in III indicate Q_3 and T_3 respectively. (2) T wave inversion in V_1 and V_2. These 2 ECG abnormalities are typical of pulmonary embolism. (Reproduced with permission. Chia BL, Tan HC, Lim YT. Right sided chest lead ECG abnormalities in acute pulmonary embolism. Int J Cardiol 1997; 61: 43 [with adaptation]).

CHRONIC OBSTRUCTIVE LUNG DISEASE

In chronic obstructive lung disease such as emphysema (Fig. 3.13), the following ECG abnormalities are seen:

(1) P wave axis > 80° in the frontal plane (2) "P pulmonale" (3) Right axis deviation (4) Clockwise rotation of the heart round its longitudinal axis, resulting in rS complexes in leads V_1 to V_5/V_6 (5) Low QRS voltages especially in the limb leads and also in the left praecordial leads. (6) "Lead 1" sign, which is reflected by an isoelectric P wave, a QRS amplitude < +1.5 mm and a T wave amplitude < +0.05 mm (all in lead I) (7) Importantly, although right ventricular hypertrophy is present anatomically, tall R waves are not seen in V_1 unlike other examples of right ventricular hypertrophy (Figs. 3.9 and 3.10).

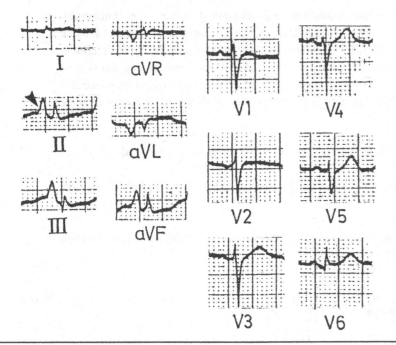

Fig. 3.13 Chronic obstructive lung disease. Note: (1) Vertical P wave axis in the frontal plane (approximately +90°). (2) **"P pulmonale"**. This is best seen in II, III and aVF. The P wave in II is peaked and measures 5 mm in height (arrowhead) indicating right atrial enlargement. (3) Clockwise rotation of the heart round its longitudinal axis resulting in rS complexes in V_1 to V_5. (4) Low QRS voltages in the limb leads, and in V_5 and V_6. (5) "Lead I Sign".

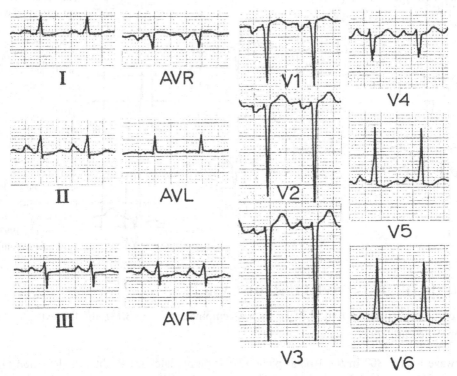

Fig. 3.14 Dilated cardiomyopathy in a middle aged man showing the **ECG-Congestive heart failure Triad**. The ECG criteria of this triad consists of: (1) Low QRS voltages (≤ 8 mm) in all the 6 limb leads (2) Prominent QRS complexes in the praecordial leads (S V_1/V_2 + R V_5/V_6 = ≥ 35 mm) and (3) Poor R wave progression from V_1 to V_4. The ECG in our patient fulfills these criteria showing: (1) The voltages of all the QRS complexes in the limb leads are < 8 mm (2) S V_2 + RV_5 = 45 mm. (3) Poor r wave progression from V_1 to V_4. This ECG pattern is a specific but not sensitive indicator of severe systolic heart failure of varying aetiologies.

CARDIOMYOPATHY

There are many ECG abnormalities associated with the cardiomyopathies. In **hypertrophic cardiomyopathy**, the commonest ECG changes are left ventricular hypertrophy, T wave inversion (Fig. 3.16) and pathological Q waves which are usually seen in the inferolateral leads (Fig. 3.15). Occasionally, a giant T wave inversion is seen and this is highly suggestive of apical hypertrophic cardiomyopathy.

In **dilated cardiomyopathy**, left ventricular hypertrophy, deep pathogical Q waves, left atrial enlargement (Fig. 3.14), and left bundle branch block (complete and incomplete) are all features of this condition. In some cases, the QRS voltages in the limb leads may be decreased although they are increased in the praecordial leads (Fig. 3.14).

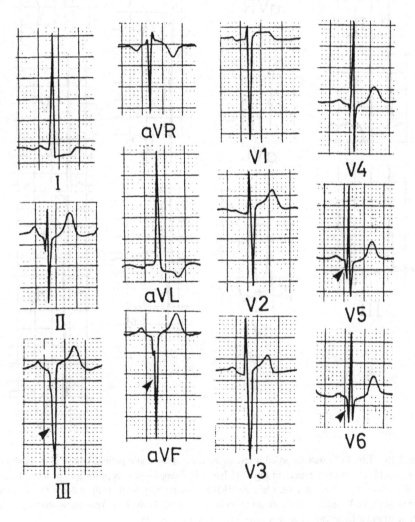

Fig. 3.15 Hypertrophic cardiomyopathy. ECG of a 26-year-old woman with hypertrophic cardiomyopathy which was confirmed by two-dimensional echocardiography. Note: pathological Q waves in III, aVF, V_5 and V_6 (arrowheads). The Q waves in III and aVF are extremely deep and "dagger like".

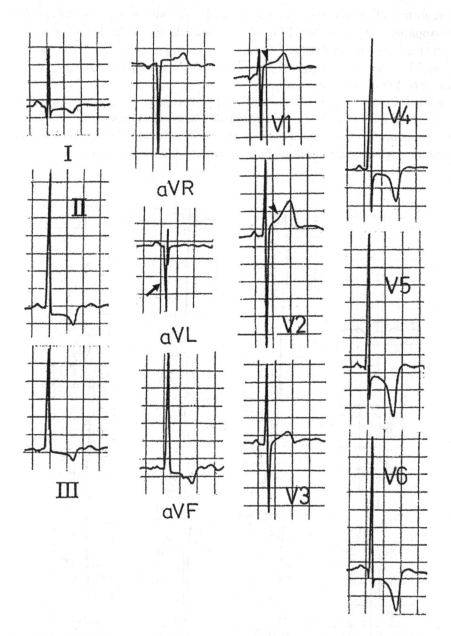

Fig. 3.16 This ECG was recorded a few years later in the same patient whose ECG is shown in Fig. 3.15. The deep Q waves in Fig. 3.15 have all disappeared except for a new deep Q wave in aVL (arrow). Instead, a severe left ventricular hypertrophy with strain pattern has evolved. Arrowheads in V_1 and V_2 indicate an elevated ST segment which is frequently seen in severe left ventricular hypertrophy and is often mistaken for a STEMI.

INTRACRANIAL HAEMORRHAGE

Some of the most bizarre ECG changes are seen in patients with subarachnoid and intracranial haemorrhage. These include deeply inverted and wide T waves or less commonly, prominent, upright T waves in the praecordial leads. The QT interval is also markedly prolonged (Fig. 3.17).

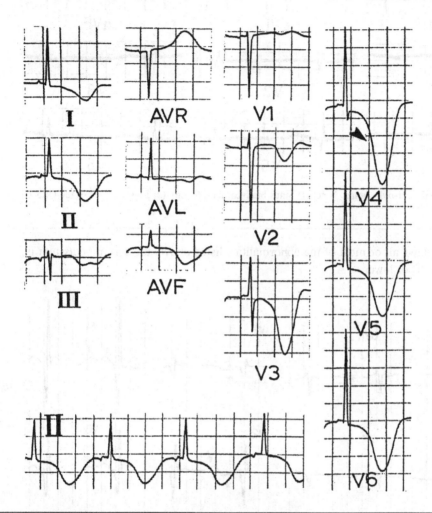

Fig. 3.17 ECG was recorded in a 75-year-old woman with proven **subarachnoid haemorrhage**. Note: (1) T waves which are very deeply inverted and very wide in multiple leads but especially in V_3 to V_6 (arrowhead in V_4). (2) The QTc interval (0.69 sec) is markedly prolonged. (3) The P waves are flat and abnormal looking indicating that they are most likely atrial in origin and the PR interval is very short (approximately 0.08 sec).

MYXOEDEMA

In myxoedema (Fig. 3.18), the following changes are seen: (1) Sinus bradycardia (2) Widespread decrease in the voltages of the QRS complexes (3) Flat or inverted T waves.

HYPOKALAEMIA

The ECG is a useful tool for the diagnosis of both hypokalaemia and hyperkalaemia. As the serum potassium falls, the U wave becomes taller and T wave becomes flatter. Therefore, an accurate sign of hypokalaemia is a U wave equal to or taller than the T wave in the same lead (Fig. 3.19). In severe hypokalaemia, very prominent U waves are seen together with T wave inversion and slight ST segment depression. In a few leads, the T and U waves may merge forming wide TU complexes and prolonged QTU intervals. First and second degree (Wenckebach phenomenon) AV block, ventricular ectopic beats and other ventricular arrhythmias can also be seen in hypokalaemia.

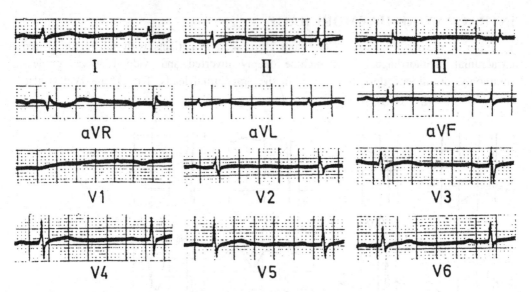

Fig. 3.18 **Myxoedema** in a 62-year-old woman. Note: (1) Sinus bradycardia (56/min). (2) Low voltages of the QRS complexes. (3) Flat or isoelectric T waves.

If the ECG shows all or most of the abnormalities listed above, the serum potassium is often < 2.7 mmol/L or lower.

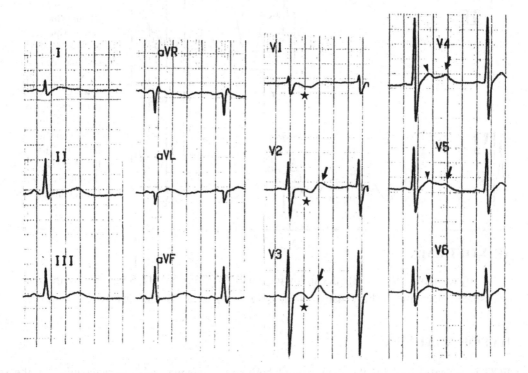

Fig. 3.19 **Severe hypokalaemia** (serum potassium = 1.6 mmol/L) in a 23-year-old man with thyrotoxic periodic paralysis who presented with weakness in all 4 limbs. Note: (1) Tall U waves (arrows) in multiple leads. In some leads (e.g. V_2, V_3), the U waves are very prominent (4 mm in V_3). (2) The T waves in V_4, V_5 and V_6 (arrowheads) are flat. In V_4, the T wave and the U wave are approximately equal in amplitude. (3) T wave inversion is seen from V_1 to V_3 (asterisk). (4) In II, III and aVF, the T and U waves have merged to form wide TU complexes. The QTU interval (0.66 sec) is markedly prolonged (ECG courtesy of Professor Jin-Seng Cheah).

HYPERKALAEMIA

The main ECG abnormality in hyperkalaemia is the presence of tall T waves with no ST segment elevation. Very tall T waves are also a hallmark of the early repolarization pattern; but here unlike in hyperkalaemia, there is ST segment elevation. Just as important as the height of the T wave in hyperkalaemia is its unique morphology. The T waves are not only tall, but their bases are narrow and they are also slender, symmetrical, and peaked. With further elevation of the serum potassium, the P waves disappear and this is followed by widening of the QRS complexes accompanied by slowing of the ventricular rate.

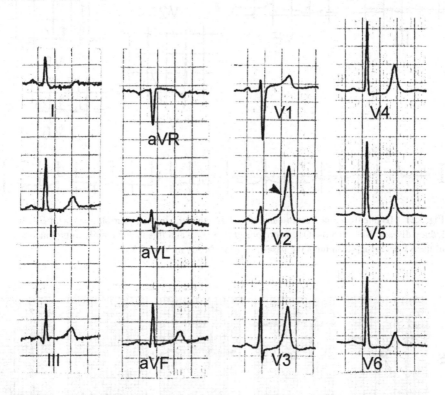

Fig. 3.20 Hyperkalaemia (serum potassium = 8.1 mmol/L) in a 53-year-old woman with chronic kidney disease. Note that the T waves (arrowhead) are not only tall in V_2 and V_3 (15 mm in V_2), but are also unique in their morphology. Their bases are narrow and they are slender, symmetrical and peaked. This unique T wave morphology is also seen in V_4, even though the amplitude of the T wave in this lead is not increased.

HYPOCALCAEMIA AND HYPERCALCAEMIA

In hypocalcaemia, the QTc interval is prolonged and this is due mainly to lengthening of the ST segment which hugs the baseline (Fig. 3.21). In hypercalcaemia, the QTc interval is shortened.

JUVENILE ECG PATTERN

T wave inversion in leads V_1 to V_4 is usually present in the child (Fig. 3.22). After about 14 years of age, T wave inversion is common in lead V_1 and is sometimes accompanied by T wave inversion in lead V_2. However, isolated T wave inversion in lead V_2 is abnormal.

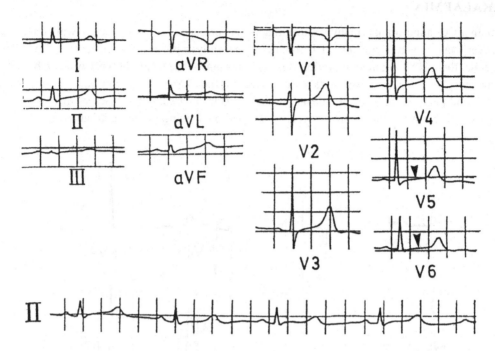

Fig. 3.21 Hypocalcaemia (serum calcium = 1.71 mmol/L) in a 52-year-old man with chronic kidney disease. Note that the QTc is prolonged (0.51 sec) and this is due mainly to prolongation of the ST segment which hugs the base-line (arrowheads in V_5 and V_6).

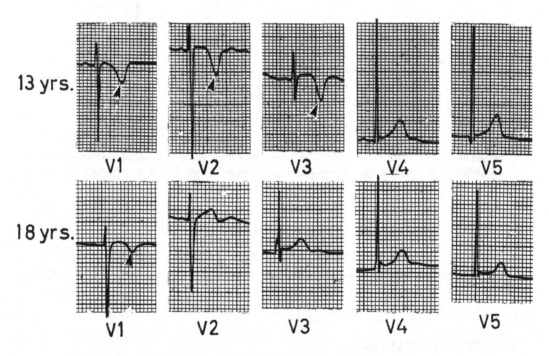

Fig. 3.22 Juvenile ECG pattern. Top panel, which was recorded when the male individual was 13 years old, shows deep T wave inversion in V_1 to V_3 (arrowheads). Bottom panel was recorded when he was 18 years old and shows disappearance of the T wave inversion except in V_1 (arrowhead).

ATHLETE'S HEART

In highly trained athletes, certain ECG changes are commonly seen. These include sinus bradycardia, first degree AV block and Mobitz Type 1 second degree AV block (Wenckebach phenomenon), increase in QRS voltages, incomplete right bundle branch block and early repolarization pattern. Unlike in the past, where prominent T wave inversion was considered as part of the athlete's heart syndrome, the opinion today is that > 1 mm T wave inversion, ≥ 0.5 mm ST segment depression and pathological Q waves (occurring in ≥ 2 contiguous leads) should all not be present.

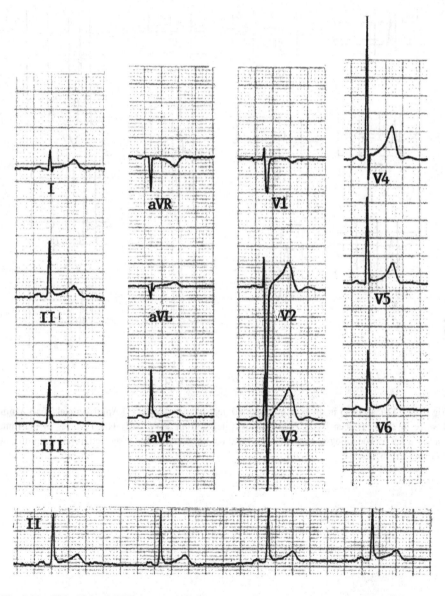

Fig. 3.23 This 12-lead ECG was recorded in a young man who was a national football (soccer) player. It shows: (1) Sinus bradycardia (47/min). (2) The amplitudes of the QRS complexes are markedly increased. S in V_2 = 35 mm and R in V_4 = 40 mm. Both these features are commonly seen in the **Athlete's Heart Syndrome**. (ECG courtesy of Assistant Professor Khim-Leng Tong).

FLAT OR INVERTED T WAVES (see page 36)

Flat or mildly inverted T waves often cause confusion as to their significance. Although ischaemic heart disease is frequently suspected, it is important to remember that such T wave changes are non-specific. Apart from ischaemic heart disease, mild T wave inversion may be seen in normal individuals (Fig. 3.24), in mitral valve prolapse, and also in many other situations such as hyperventilation, change in posture, drinking ice water, eating and emotional upset.

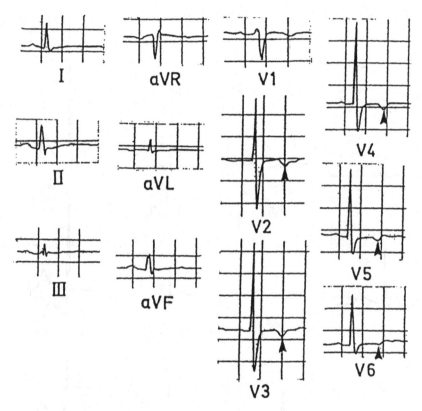

Fig. 3.24 12-lead ECG in an asymptomatic 60-year-old man. Note: (1) Approximately 1 to 2 mm T wave inversion is seen from V_1 to V_6 (arrowheads from V_2-V_6). (2) The T waves in the limb leads are flat. Echocardiography was normal and coronary angiography showed minor insignificant coronary artery disease.

ISOLATED Q III

Occasionally, the presence of a prominent Q wave in only limb lead III (Q III) poses a dilemma as to its diagnostic significance. Such a finding may be seen in normal people, but is also seen in old inferior myocardial infarction and acute pulmonary embolism. The Q III is likely to be abnormal if it is wide or if Q waves are also present in leads aVF and II. Although disappearance or diminution of the Q wave in inspiration is a point in favour of it being benign, organic cardiac disease cannot be completely excluded as illustrated in Fig. 3.25.

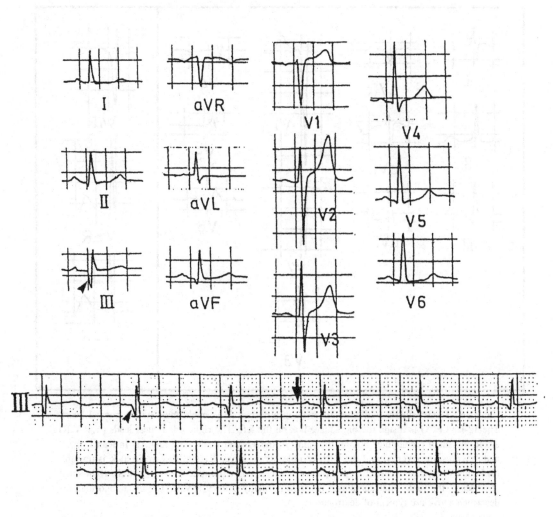

Fig. 3.25 ECG of a 60-year-old asymptomatic man showing a deep and wide pathological Q wave which is present only in III (arrowhead). The top and bottom panels of the rhythm strip (recorded in lead III) are continuous. Arrow indicates the beginning of deep inspiration which has resulted in a disappearance of the Q wave (arrowhead). Two-dimensional echocardiography shows hypokinesia of the inferior wall of the left ventricle, due most likely to a previous silent inferior myocardial infarction.

DEXTROCARDIA

In the presence of dextrocardia with situs inversus, the ECG in the limb leads look similar to a tracing where the right and left arm leads have been reversed. This condition should be strongly suspected if the P wave is inverted in lead I. Other ECG abnormalities include a negative QRS complex and an inverted T wave in lead I and a positive P wave in lead aVR. Leads V_1 to V_6 show regression of the QRS complexes. However, in the right sided chest leads, the QRS complexes progress normally from lead V_3R to V_6R (Fig. 3.26).

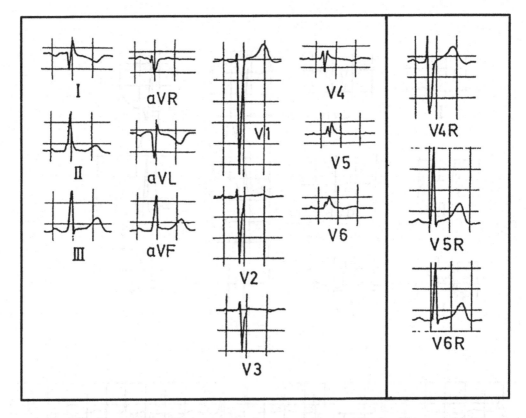

Fig. 3.26 **Dextrocardia** with situs inversus in a normal 17-year-old male with a normal heart. The 12-lead ECG is inside the big square box on the left. The right-sided chest leads (V_4R-V_6R) are in the small rectangular box on the right. In the 12-lead ECG, note that: (1) In lead I, the P and T waves are inverted and the QRS complex is negative. (2) The P wave in aVR is upright. (3) Leads V_1-V_6 show ventricular complexes of decreasing amplitude. However, in the right-sided chest leads, the ventricular complexes progress normally from V_4R-V_6R. The ECG abnormalities described above are typical of dextrocardia.

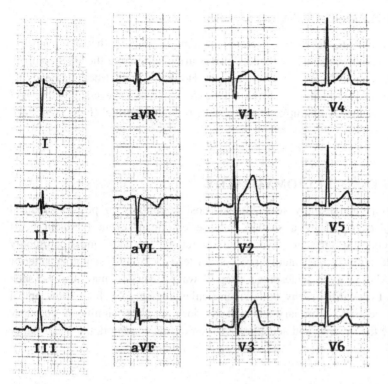

Fig. 3.27 12-lead ECG recorded with reversal of the right and left arm leads in a 30-year-old normal man. The limb lead abnormalities are identical to that seen in dextrocardia: (1) an inverted P wave, negative QRS complex and an inverted T wave in I and (2) a positive P wave in aVR. However, unlike dextrocardia, the QRS complexes in the chest (V) leads are all normal (see text in page 70).

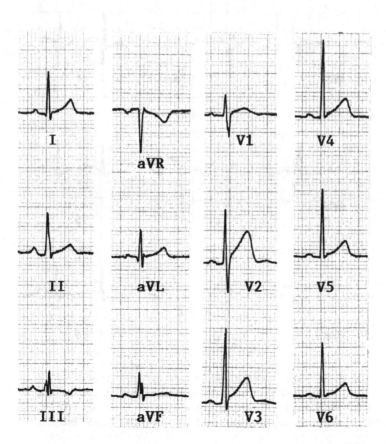

Fig. 3.28 Repeat ECG recorded from the same patient whose ECG is shown in Fig. 3.27, now with the arm leads in the correct position. The 12-lead ECG is now completely normal.

REVERSAL of RIGHT and LEFT ARM LEADS

When the right and left arm leads are reversed, the abnormalities in the limb leads are identical to that seen in dextrocardia. The P and T waves are inverted and the QRS complex is negative in lead I. In lead aVR, the P wave is upright. However, in dextrocardia, leads V_1 to V_6 show ventricular complexes of decreasing amplitude, whereas in reversal of the right and left arm leads, the ventricular complexes in leads V_1 to V_6 are normal (Figs. 3.26, 3.27, 3.28).

TAKOTSUBO (STRESS) CARDIOMYOPATHY

This entity, which is increasingly seen, occurs most commonly in post-menopausal women. It is usually triggered by a sudden, intense emotional event ("broken heart syndrome") and presents like an acute myocardial infarction. The ECG most commonly shows ST segment elevation in the anterior praecordial leads, closely resembling anterior STEMI (Fig. 3.29). Alternatively, widespread deep T wave inversion may also be seen simulating NSTEMI. Echocardiography or left ventricular angiography both show apical ballooning of the left ventricle. Coronary angiography does not show significant coronary artery disease. Despite the severity and acute presentation of this condition, the abnormality is often transient.

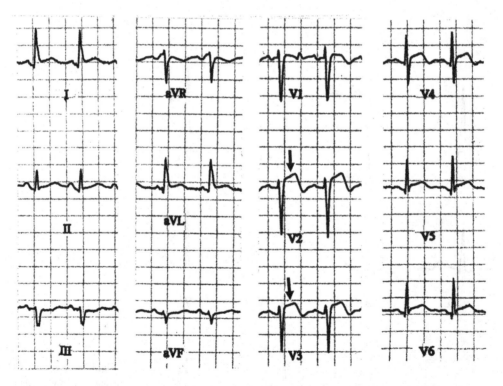

Fig. 3.29   12-lead ECG of a 54-year-woman with **Takotsubo Cardiomyopathy**. There is 1-3 mm ST segment elevation in V_1 to V_6, I and aVL (arrows in V_2 and V_3). In addition, there are also biphasic T waves from V_2 to V_4. (Reproduced with permission. Kuntjoro I, Teo SG, Poh KK. Nonischaemic causes of ST segment elevation. Singapore Med J 2012; 53(6): 367 [with adaptation]).

NORMAL VARIANT IN YOUNG BLACK MALES

In about 4% of young normal black males, ST segment elevation in combination with T wave inversion is seen in the mid-praecordial leads.

OBESITY

The majority of obese patients without heart disease have normal ECGs. In a study of 1,029 subjects, low QRS voltage was seen in only 3.9% of the subjects. (Frank S et al. J Am Coll Cardiol 1986; 2: 295).

HYPOTHERMIA

Patients with hypothermia may develop a distinctive ECG pattern in which a humplike elevation is usually localized to the junction of the end of the QRS complex and the beginning of the ST segment (J point). These pathological J waves are called Osborn Waves (Fig. 3.30). Other ECG abnormalities in hypothermia include sinus bradycardia, prolonged PR and QT intervals, T wave inversion and atrial fibrillation.

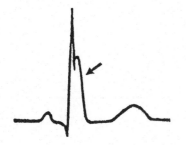

Fig. 3.30 Hypothermia. Arrow indicates humplike elevation called **Osborn Wave**.

THYROTOXICOSIS

The most common ECG changes in thyrotoxicosis are sinus tachycardia and an increase in voltage of the QRS, P and T wave complexes. Atrial fibrillation is seen in about 10-20% of all cases.

ARTIFACTS

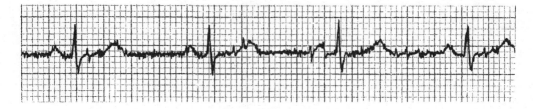

Fig. 3.31 ECG (lead II) was taken from a 12-lead ECG which was recorded from a patient who was not relaxed. The baseline is not clear because it has been replaced by sharp and irregular spikes.

CHAPTER 4

CARDIAC ARRHYTHMIAS

INTRODUCTION

Cardiac arrhythmias are frequently encountered in clinical practice. They must be diagnosed and carefully evaluated, especially as to their significance and whether treatment is required or not.

ASSESSMENT

Two principles are of paramount importance:

(1) **An accurate diagnosis of the cardiac arrhythmia must be made**. This is because different arrhythmias frequently have markedly different clinical significance. For example, a patient presenting with a regular tachycardia of about 170/min may have either supraventricular or ventricular tachycardia. Both these arrhythmias have vastly different prognostic implications and require different therapeutic approaches. Although the clinical history and examination may provide clues about the arrhythmia, an ECG is necessary for precise definition. A 12-lead ECG together with a long "rhythm strip", usually recorded in either leads II or V_1, is invaluable.

Identifying P waves is crucial because the temporal relationship of the P and QRS complexes often is the key to the exact diagnosis of the type of arrhythmia present. If P waves are not clearly identifiable, the oesophageal lead ECG (i.e. ECG recorded from an electrode placed in the oesophagus) can be done. P waves are greatly magnified in the oesophageal lead ECG and are therefore clearly visible (Fig. 4.1). However, because of the inconvenience of this technique, it is today seldom performed.

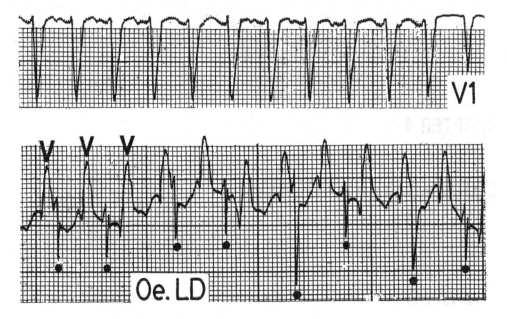

Fig. 4.1 Top panel shows ventricular tachycardia. There are no clearly visible P waves. Bottom panel was recorded at the same time as the top panel using an oesophageal lead (Oe. LD). Note that large, biphasic P waves (closed circles) are clearly seen. The ventricular complexes are labelled V.

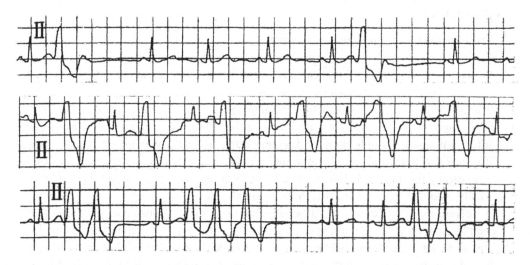

Fig. 4.2 **24-hour Holter monitor recording** in a patient who complained of palpitations. The top, middle and bottom panels were recorded at different times of the day. Top panel shows frequent, uniform ventricular ectopic beats, middle panel ventricular bigeminy and bottom panel ventricular ectopic beats occurring in pairs and in 3 consecutive beats.

Since cardiac arrhythmias are often intermittent, they may not be detected in a routine recording of the 12-lead ECG. **Twenty four hour Holter monitor recording** is indicated if an arrhythmia is suspected but not confirmed in the routine ECG (Fig. 4.2). **Exercise stress test** can also be used to detect cardiac arrhythmias. In patients with infrequent symptoms, event recorders are useful. In selected cases, an **electrophysiology test** is indicated especially in: (a) Cases of supraventricular tachycardia which are resistant to conventional pharmacological therapy (b) Patients with sustained ventricular tachycardia or ventricular fibrillation in the absence of an acute myocardial infarction and (c) Patients presenting with syncopal episodes who are suspected to have third degree (complete) atrioventricular (AV) block or sinus arrest, but whose resting ECG or 24-hour Holter monitor recording fail to confirm these arrhythmias. In patients presenting with syncope, **a tilt-table** test is also useful.

(2) The clinical setting in which a cardiac arrhythmia occurs is very important, especially in deciding whether treatment is necessary or not. For example, frequent ventricular ectopic beats in a person with a structurally normal heart are benign and do not require treatment except when there are distressing symptoms, such as palpitations. In an opposite situation, a patient with a significantly impaired left ventricular function (e.g. left ventricular ejection fraction < 30%) due to chronic myocardial disease or some other structural heart disease, associated with frequent ventricular ectopic beats will have an increase risk of ventricular fibrillation.

CLINICAL PRESENTATION

The commonest clinical presentation of cardiac arrhythmias is **palpitation**, which is usually caused by ventricular/atrial ectopic beats, atrial fibrillation, supraventricular tachycardia or ventricular tachycardia. Prolonged episodes of supraventricular tachycardia or atrial fibrillation with a rapid ventricular rate, especially in the background of heart disease, may lead to congestive heart failure or hypotension. Severe bradycardia, which may be seen in third degree (complete) AV block or the sick sinus syndrome, often results in giddiness, syncope or heart failure. Ventricular fibrillation, if uncorrected, will inevitably result in death. Indeed, the most common cause of sudden cardiac death is ventricular fibrillation. However, it is important to realize that many individuals with cardiac arrhythmias (e.g. ventricular ectopic beats) are asymptomatic and are unaware of their cardiac rhythm abnormalities.

AETIOLOGY

In every patient with a cardiac arrhythmia, a possible aetiology should always be sought for by a careful history, clinical examination, resting 12-lead ECG and chest X-ray. In selected cases, more sophisticated investigations which have been listed in page 15 may be indicated. However, it is important to realize that in a significant number of cases, no cause may be found despite detailed investigations.

MANAGEMENT

In many patients with cardiac arrhythmias, specific treatment may not be necessary. However, if treatment is required, one or more of the following therapeutic approaches may be employed:

(1) Physiological
  (a) Carotid sinus massage
  (b) Valsalva manoeuvre

(2) Pharmacological
  The following drugs are used in the treatment of cardiac arrhythmias:
  (a) Adenosine, digoxin and atropine
  (b) Class I antiarrhythmic drugs such as procaineamide (Ia), lignocaine (Ib), propafenone and flecainide (both Ic)
  (c) Class II drugs which are the beta-blockers
  (d) Class III drugs such as amiodarone and sotalol. Sotalol also has beta-blocker property
  (e) Class IV drugs such as verapamil and diltiazem

(3) Electrical
  (a) Cardioversion (b) Cardiac pacing (c) Radiofrequency catheter ablation
  (d) Implantable cardioverter-defibrillator.

Although many of the more potent antiarrhythmic drugs (e.g. Class Ic drugs such as flecainide) are extremely effective in suppressing cardiac arrhythmias, they are paradoxically also potentially proarrhythmic (i.e. they may aggravate preexisting arrhythmias or induce new arrhythmias), especially in patients with significant structural heart disease.

Most of the supraventricular tachycardias and atrial flutter cases are amenable to curative radiofrequency ablation with a high success rate and a low complication risk. Patients at high risk of sudden cardiac death (e.g. resuscitated cardiac arrest survivor) benefit greatly from treatment with an implantable cardioverter defibrillator, in the absence of a reversible cause for the initial episode of ventricular fibrillation.

CHAPTER 5

SUPRAVENTRICULAR ARRHYTHMIAS

CLASSIFICATION OF CARDIAC ARRHYTHMIAS

Table 5.1 is a simple classification of the cardiac arrhythmias.

TABLE 5.1

CLASSIFICATION OF CARDIAC ARRHYTHMIAS
SUPRAVENTRICULAR
Sinus tachycardia
Sinus bradycardia
Sinus arrhythmia
Sinoatrial block
Sinus arrest
Junctional (nodal) rhythm
Junctional (nodal) escape beats
Wandering pacemaker
Supraventricular ectopic beats
Supraventricular tachycardia
Multifocal atrial tachycardia
Accelerated junctional rhythm
Atrial fibrillation
Atrial flutter
Wolff-Parkinson-White Syndrome
VENTRICULAR
Ventricular ectopic beats
Ventricular tachycardia (monomorphic and polymorphic)
"Torsades de Pointes"
Accelerated idioventricular rhythm
Ventricular flutter
Ventricular fibrillation
Idioventricular rhythm
Ventricular asystole
BUNDLE BRANCH BLOCK AND ATRIOVENTRICULAR (AV) BLOCK
Right and left bundle branch block
Left anterior and left posterior hemiblock
First, second and third degree AV block

THE NORMAL CARDIAC RHYTHM

Normally, the cardiac impulse arises from the sinoatrial node and the resting heart rate is around 70/min. In sinus tachycardia, the sinus rate exceeds 100/min and in sinus bradycardia, it is slower than 60/min.

(1) SINUS TACHYCARDIA

Sinus tachycardia is a normal physiological response to exercise. When it occurs at rest there may be an underlying condition such as anxiety, heart failure, fever or thyrotoxicosis. The ECG shows regular, normal P waves which usually exceed 100 to 140/min (Fig. 5.1).

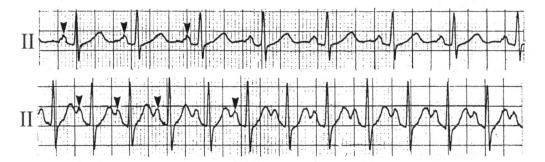

Fig. 5.1 Sinus tachycardia. The ECG was recorded in a 30-year-old woman during treadmill exercise stress test. The top panel was recorded at rest and shows a sinus rate of around 88/min. The bottom panel was recorded in the recovery period soon after termination of exercise and it shows a sinus tachycardia of around 149/min. **Arrowheads in this ECG and in all other subsequent ECGs in Chapters 5, 6 and 7 indicate sinus P waves unless stated otherwise.**

> **Arrowheads in Fig. 5.1 and in all other subsequent ECGs in Chapters 5, 6 and 7 indicate sinus P waves unless stated otherwise.**

(2) SINUS BRADYCARDIA

Sinus bradycardia is common and may be found in health as well as in disease. The ECG shows normal P waves which are less than 60/min (Fig. 5.2). Physically fit individuals and athletes usually have slow resting heart rates of around 40 to 60/min due to a high degree of vagotonia. Sinus bradycardia may also be due to beta-blocker therapy.

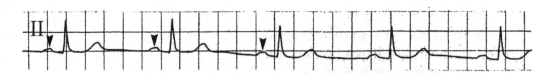

Fig. 5.2 Sinus bradycardia. ECG of a 66-year-old man with previous myocardial infarction. The sinus bradycardia of around 53/min is due to beta-blocker therapy.

(3) SINUS ARRHYTHMIA

In this arrhythmia, the sinus rate increases with inspiration and decreases with expiration (Fig. 5.3). Sinus arrhythmia is often a normal physiological phenomenon and is particularly accentuated in infants and young children.

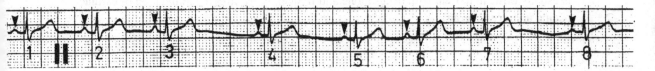

Fig. 5.3 Sinus arrhythmia. There is marked variation in the sinus rate as it increases with inspiration (beats 1, 2, 3, 6 and 7) and decreases with expiration (beats 4, 5 and 8).

(4) SINOATRIAL BLOCK

In sinoatrial block, there is sudden failure of either the sinoatrial node to discharge or the sinus impulse to be conducted to the atrium, resulting in absence of the P wave in the ECG (Fig. 5.4). The P–P intervals of the long pauses are multiples of the normal sinus cycle. For example, in a 2:1 or a 3:1 sinoatrial block, they are twice or three times the normal sinus cycle respectively. Sinoatrial block may be due to the sick sinus syndrome, digitalis intoxication, acute myocarditis or acute myocardial infarction. No specific treatment is required if the pauses are of short duration or if the patient is asymptomatic. However, if the pauses are long and especially if they are associated with syncope, cardiac pacing is indicated.

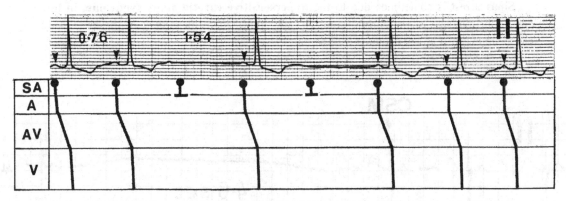

Fig. 5.4 2:1 sinoatrial block. The time interval is approximately 0.76 sec between the first and second, fourth and fifth and fifth and sixth P waves and approximately 1.54 sec between the second and third and third and fourth P waves. The longer intervals are double the shorter intervals indicating a 2:1 sinoatrial block. **The following abbreviations are used in this and all subsequent laddergrams in Chapters 5, 6 and 7. SA = sinoatrial node, A = atrium, AV = atrioventricular node, V = ventricles.**

> **The following abbreviations are used in the laddergram shown in Fig. 5.4 and in all subsequent laddergrams in Chapters 5, 6 and 7. SA = sinoatrial node, A = atrium, AV = atrioventricular node, V = ventricles.**

Patients with the **sick sinus syndrome** may present with a wide variety of arrhythmias such as severe sinus bradycardia, sinoatrial block, and sinus arrest. In the "alternating bradycardia-tachycardia syndrome", which is another presentation of the sick sinus syndrome, periods of marked sinus bradycardia or **sinus arrest** alternate with episodes of rapid supraventricular tachycardia, atrial fibrillation or atrial flutter (Fig. 5.5). This condition is usually difficult to treat with drugs alone and frequently requires a combination of cardiac pacing and drug therapy.

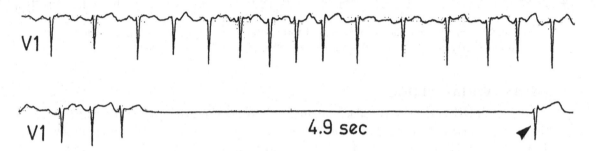

Fig. 5.5 Alternating bradycardia-tachycardia syndrome in a 62-year-old woman who complained of syncope. The top and bottom ECG strips (non-continuous) are taken from a 24-hour Holter monitor recording. The top strip shows atrial fibrillation with a rapid ventricular rate. The bottom strip shows spontaneous termination of the atrial fibrillation. This is followed by a pause of about 4.9 sec due to sinus arrest. Arrowhead indicates a junctional escape beat.

Sinus arrest is sometimes due to the **hypersensitive carotid sinus syndrome**. In this condition, massage of the carotid sinus, or sometimes mere movement of the head, may cause sinus arrest and syncope (Fig. 5.6).

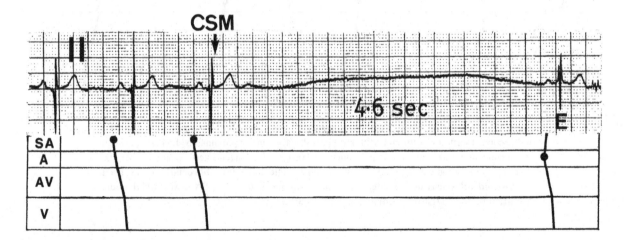

Fig. 5.6 Hypersensitive carotid sinus syndrome in a 64-year-old man who presented with recurrent syncope. ECG shows: (1) A pause of 4.6 sec due to sinus arrest induced by gentle carotid sinus massage (CSM) (2) E is an escape beat, probably atrial in origin.

(6) JUNCTIONAL (NODAL) ESCAPE BEAT

In patients with sinus bradycardia, sinoatrial block or sinus arrest, the depression or absence of sinus activity may allow the emergence of a subsidiary pacemaker in either the atria, AV junction or the ventricles, resulting in what is termed an escape beat (Fig. 5.7).

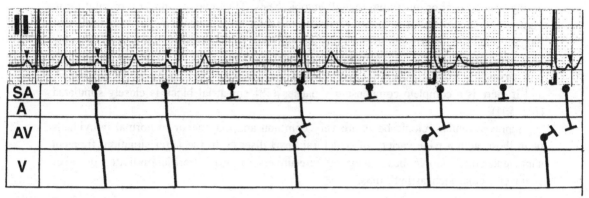

Fig. 5.7 Junctional escape beat. Note: (1) The interval between the third and fourth, fourth and fifth and fifth and sixth P waves is double the interval between the first and second and the second and third P waves, indicating a 2:1 sinoatrial block. (2) Junctional escape beats (J). (3) AV dissociation.

(7) WANDERING PACEMAKER

In this arrhythmia which is frequently associated with sinus bradycardia, multiple atrial escape beats are seen (Fig. 5.8). Wandering pacemaker is a benign arrhythmia and is commonly seen in normal individuals.

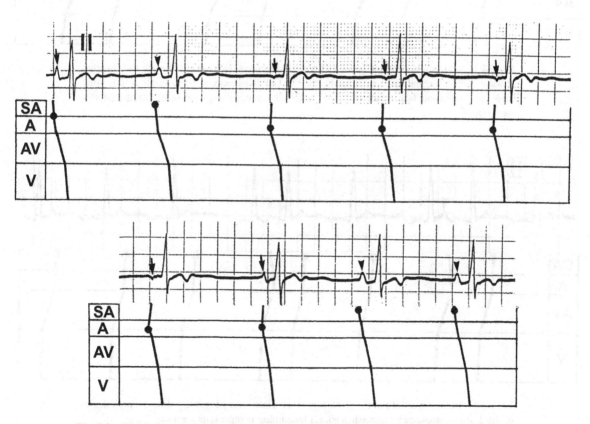

Fig. 5.8 Wandering pacemaker. Top and bottom panels are continuous. Arrowheads indicate sinus P waves and arrows indicate atrial escape beats.

(8) SUPRAVENTRICULAR ECTOPIC BEATS

Supraventricular ectopic beats may arise in either the atrium or the AV node junction, giving rise to atrial or junctional (nodal) ectopic beats. They may be uniform or multiform. Figure 5.9 shows uniform supraventricular ectopic beats occurring in bigeminy and Fig. 5.10 shows multiform supraventricular ectopic beats. A supraventricular ectopic beat may be conducted normally or with aberrant ventricular conduction (Fig. 6.3), a phenomenon which is discussed in Chapter 6. A very premature supraventricular ectopic beat may not be conducted, and if there is a complete compensatory pause, a 2:1 sinoatrial block is closely simulated (Fig. 5.11).

Supraventricular ectopic beats are very common and may occur in normal individuals or in those with a wide variety of structural heart disease. In the latter situation, frequent supraventricular ectopic beats may be forerunners of atrial fibrillation/flutter or other supraventricular tachyarrhythmias.

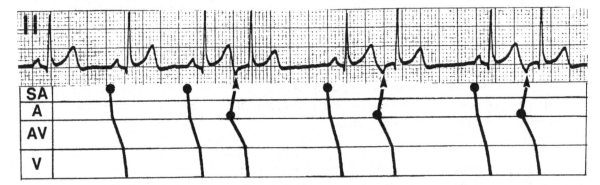

Fig. 5.9 Uniform atrial ectopic beats occurring in bigeminy. Note: (1) Premature and inverted P waves which are indicated by arrowheads. (2) The atrial ectopic beats occur in bigeminy after the first ectopic beat – rule of bigeminy. (3) The compensatory pause is almost complete (see page 97).

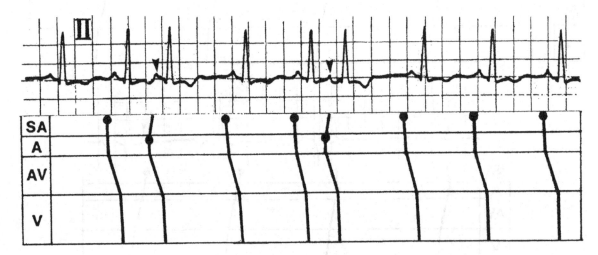

Fig. 5.10 Multiform atrial ectopic beats. Note: (1) Different coupling intervals and morphologies of the 2 atrial ectopic beats (arrowheads). (2) Incomplete compensatory pause.

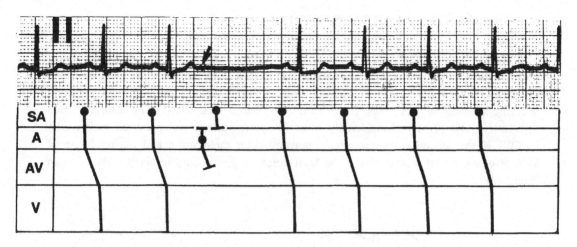

Fig. 5.11 Blocked atrial ectopic beat (arrow). Note complete compensatory pause. 2.1 sinoatrial block may be misdiagnosed if the blocked atrial ectopic beat is not recognized.

(9) MULTIFOCAL ATRIAL TACHYCARDIA

In this arrhythmia, normal sinus rhythm is replaced by a variety of atrial beats. The following features distinguish multifocal atrial tachycardia from multiform atrial ectopic beats: (1) P waves of at least 3 different morphologies; (2) Varying P–P intervals; (3) Varying P–R intervals; and (4) Absence of a dominant pacemaker (5) Atrial rate $\geq$ 100/min (Fig. 5.12). The commonest cause of multifocal atrial tachycardia is chronic obstructive lung disease.

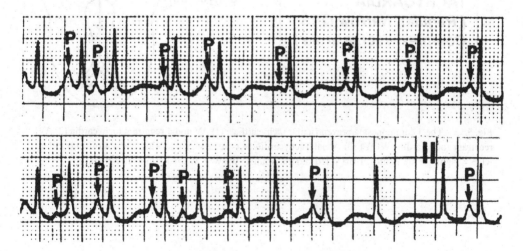

Fig. 5.12 Multifocal atrial tachycardia in a 71-year-old man with heart failure. Top and bottom panels are continuous. Note: (1) P waves of multiple morphologies (arrows). (2) Varying P–P intervals. (3) Varying PR intervals. (4) Absence of a dominant pacemaker. (5) Atrial tachycardia ($\geq$ 100/min).

(10) SUPRAVENTRICULAR TACHYCARDIA

Supraventricular tachycardia is an important cause of **"Regular narrow QRS complex (< 0.12 sec) tachycardia"** and comprises three distinct entities: **(1) AV nodal reentrant tachycardia (2) AV reentrant tachycardia (associated with an accessory pathway)** and **(3) Atrial tachycardia**. Of these three, AV nodal reentrant tachycardia is the most common occuring in about 60% of cases. It can be divided into 2 varieties: (1) The common slow-fast variety and (2) The considerably rarer fast-slow variety. AV reentrant tachycardia (WPW) is the second most common supraventricular tachycardia and occurs in about 30% of cases. Atrial tachycardia is the least common and occurs in about 10% of cases (Fig. 5.13).

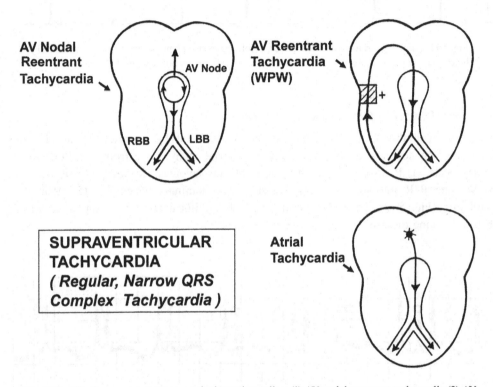

Fig. 5.13 The 3 commonest supraventricular tachycardias: (1) AV nodal reentrant tachycardia (2) AV reentrant tachycardia (WPW) (3) Atrial Tachycardia (+ = accessory pathway, AV = atrioventricular, RBB = right bundle branch, LBB = left bundle branch, WPW = Wolff-Parkinson-White).

The ECG in supraventricular tachycardia shows regular, narrow QRS complexes (< 0.12 sec) at a rate of about 170/min or more. **QRS alternans**, where the QRS complexes alternate in height, is occasionally seen (Fig. 5.21). Initial studies suggested that QRS alternans was a useful diagnostic feature of AV reentrant tachycardia (WPW). But subsequent studies suggested that QRS alternans was probably a function of a faster tachycardia and not a specific mechanism. However, its presence at slower rates (e.g. < 180/min) is suggestive of AV reentrant tachycardia. QRS alternans occuring with small voltage QRS, P wave and T wave complexes in patients with **sinus rhythm** is often diagnostic of **large pericardial effusion** with cardiac tamponade. However, QRS alternans occurring during supraventricular tachycardia has no bearing with pericardial effusion.

In **AV nodal reentrant tachycardia** of the slow-fast variety, the P waves are usually hidden because they are buried within or appear just after the QRS complexes (Fig. 5.14). In **AV reentrant tachycardia**, the P waves are often visible as they occur shortly after the QRS complexes, with the RP interval being shorter than the PR interval (Fig. 5.15). In **atrial tachycardia**, each QRS complex is preceded by a P wave which is different in morphology from the normal sinus P wave, with the RP interval being longer than the PR interval (Fig. 5.17).

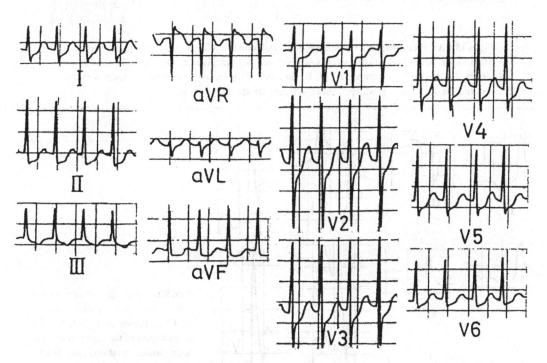

Fig. 5.14 Supraventricular **AV nodal reentrant tachycardia** in a 35-year-old woman who presented with palpitations. Note: (1) Regular, narrow QRS complex tachycardia of around 200/min. (2) No P waves are visible. (3) **Rapid upsloping ST depression** in V_2 & V_3 and **slow upsloping ST depression** in V_5, V_6 & II. Subsequent electrophysiology study confirmed that the patient was suffering from supraventricular AV nodal reentrant tachycardia.

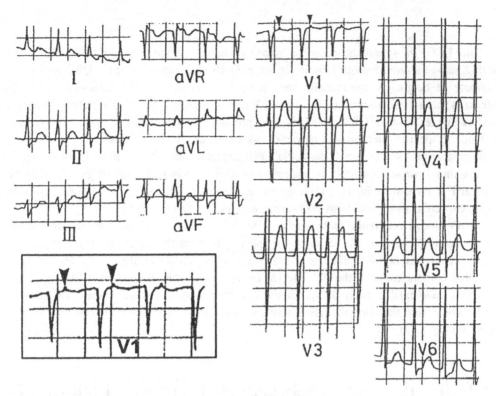

Fig. 5.15 **AV reentrant tachycardia (WPW syndrome)** in a 34-year-old man presenting with palpitations. Note: (1) Regular, narrow QRS complex tachycardia of around 166/min. (2) Clearly visible P waves in V_1 (arrowheads), II, III and aVF. They occur soon after the QRS complex resulting in a RP interval which is much shorter than the PR interval.

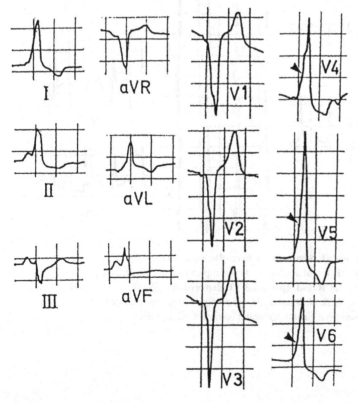

Fig. 5.16 This ECG was recorded from the same patient whose ECG is shown in Fig. 5.15 after termination of the supraventricular tachycardia. It shows the **WPW syndrome** as reflected by: (1) Short PR interval (about 0.08 sec). (2) Wide QRS complex (about 0.14 sec). (3) Delta waves in V_4, V_5, V_6 (arrowheads), I, II and aVL. The QRS complexes are negative in V_1-V_3, indicating that the WPW is Type B variety. Prominent R wave in V_5 mimics left ventricular hypertrophy.

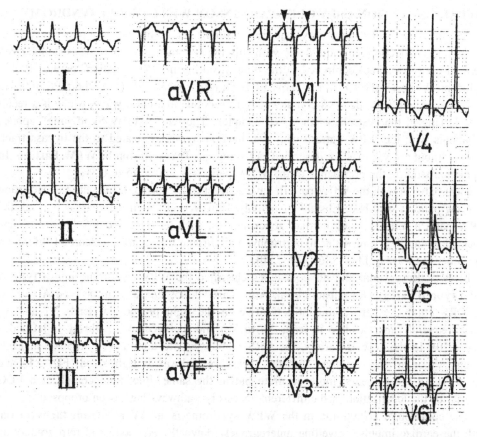

Fig. 5.17 Recurrent **atrial tachycardia** in a 2-month-old baby. Note: (1) Regular, narrow QRS complex tachycardia of around 225/min. (2) Clearly visible P waves (arrowheads in V₁) (3) RP interval equal to or longer than PR interval.

The ECG during and after an attack of supraventricular tachycardia may show ST segment depression which may persist for several hours. Although these ECG changes may mimic ischaemic heart disease, most of these patients do not have coronary artery disease. Attacks of supraventricular tachycardia may be frequent or infrequent, and each episode may be transient or prolonged. In the initial management of an acute attack of supraventricular tachycardia, a vagotonic stimulus such as carotid sinus massage or the valsalva manoeuvre is first employed. If this is unsuccessful, intravenous **adenosine** (6-12 mg) is usually given. The rate of conversion to sinus rhythm with adenosine therapy is approximately 90% with AV nodal reentrant tachycardia and AV reentrant tachycardia, but much lower in atrial tachycardia. If the supraventricular tachycardia does not respond to adenosine, or if the patient presents with hypotension or heart failure, electrical cardioversion is indicated. The need for long term prophylactic drug treatment depends largely on the frequency and the severity of the attacks. The most common drugs that are used for this purpose are AV nodal blocking agents such as **verapamil** and **beta-blockers** or **anti-arrhythmic drugs**. In AV nodal reentrant tachycardia and AV reentrant tachycardia, **radiofrequency catheter ablation** of one of the 2 pathways of the AV node or ablation of the accessory pathway respectively, is today frequently performed.

(11) PREEXCITATION and WOLFF-PARKINSON-WHTE (WPW) SYNDROME

An atrio-ventricular accessory pathway (Bundle of Kent) is a bypass tract with accelerated conduction. In individuals with this bypass tract, one ventricle is depolarized prematurely (preexcited) compared to the other resulting in "Preexcitation" or the "Wolff-Parkinson-White (WPW) Pattern". This ECG pattern consists of: (1) a short PR interval (< 0.12 sec) and (2) a wide QRS complex (≥ 0.12 sec) due to a **delta wave**, which is a result of a slurring of the upstroke of the QRS complex. The term **"WPW Syndrome"** applies to patients with the WPW pattern who also have arrhythmias related to the bypass tract. Those without arrhythmias are described as having just **Preexcitation** or **WPW Pattern**. In population studies, the prevalence of the WPW pattern is from 0.15 to 0.3%.

Most patients with the WPW pattern have a structurally normal heart with the exception of a few patients who have Ebstein's Anomaly. However, although the heart is normal, the WPW pattern mimics many cardiac abnormalities, such as right and left bundle branch block, right and left ventricular hypertrophy, and chronic transmural myocardial infarction [prominent Q waves] (Figs. 5.16, 5.19, 5.20).

In 1945, Rosenbaum and his colleagues classified the WPW syndrome into a **type A** and a **type B** variety (Rosenbaum et al. Am Heart J 1945; 29: 281). In the type A variety, the QRS complexes are dominantly positive in the right praecordial leads V_1 and V_2 (very frequently also positive in leads V_3 to V_6) and the accessory pathway is left-sided (Fig. 5.20). In the type B variety, the QRS complexes are dominantly negative in leads V_1 and V_2 or in lead V_1 alone, and the accessory pathway is right-sided (Fig. 5.16 and Fig. 5.19). In recent years, more accurate but at the same time more complicated ECG criteria for the localization of the different accessory pathways have been proposed.

The commonest arrhythmia in the WPW syndrome is an **AV reentrant tachycardia**, with the cardiac impulse travelling anterogradely down the AV node and retrogradely up the accessory pathway (Figs. 5.15, 5.21). This arrhythmia is also known as AV reentrant **orthodromic** tachycardia as opposed to the much less common AV reentrant **antidromic** tachycardia, where the impulse travels anterogradely down the accessory pathway and retrogradely up the AV node. **Atrial fibrillation** is an infrequent but a very important arrhythmia in the WPW syndrome because of it's association with sudden cardiac death. Here, the ECG shows an irregular rhythm with a very rapid ventricular rate. Most of the QRS complexes are widened, because the majority of them have been depolarized via the accessory pathway (Fig. 5.18). If the ventricular rate is very rapid, there is a significant risk of ventricular fibrillation. Drugs depressing conduction through the AV node (e.g. IV verapamil, beta-blockers, or adenosine) are contraindicated as they will result in even more impulses passing through the accessory pathway. As a result of this, the ventricular rate will be even faster, thus further increasing the risk of ventricular fibrillation. Intravenous procaineamide is the drug of choice in atrial fibrillation associated with the WPW syndrome as it blocks impulses passing through the accessory pathway. If this drug is clinically ineffective, or if the patient is hypotensive or in heart failure, electrical cardioversion should be done. When the patient is in a stable state, **ablation of the accessory pathway** is strongly indicated.

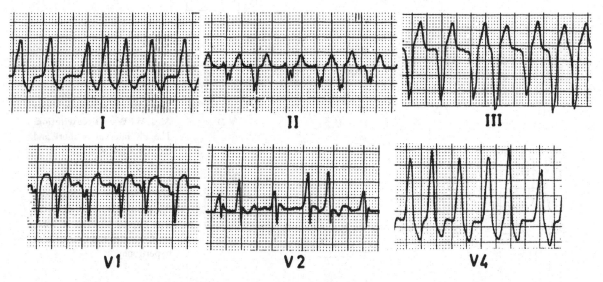

Fig. 5.18 Atrial fibrillation in a 22-year-old man with the WPW syndrome. Note: (1) Irregular rhythm and very rapid ventricular rate. (2) The QRS complexes are wide.

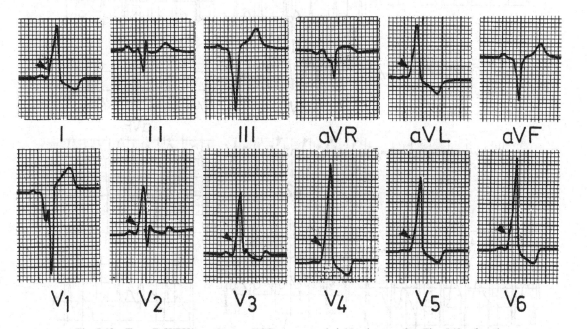

Fig. 5.19 Type B WPW syndrome. ECG was recorded 15 minutes after Fig. 5.18, after the atrial fibrillation was converted to sinus rhythm. Note: (1) Short PR interval (about 0.10 sec). (2) Delta waves in V_2 to V_6, I and aVL, (arrowheads). (3) Pathological Q waves in III, aVF and V_1, simulating old inferior myocardial infarction.

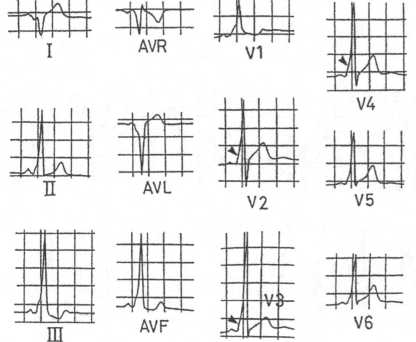

Fig. 5.20 ECG shows **Type A WPW Preexcitation**. The PR interval is short and the QRS is wide due to a delta wave (arrowheads in V_2, V_3 and V_4). The Type A WPW variety is diagnosed by positive QRS complexes from V_1 to V_6. Tall R wave in V_1 mimics right ventricular hypertrophy.

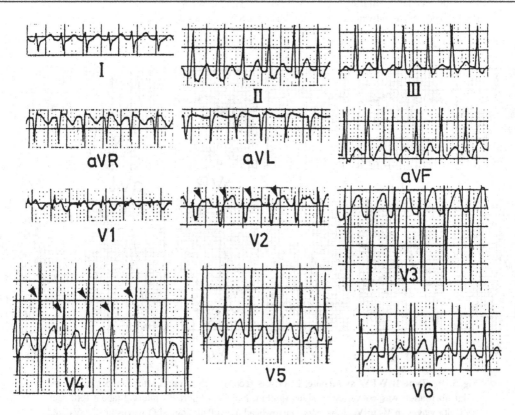

Fig. 5.21 Supraventricular tachycardia in a 16-year-old man. Note: (1) Regular, narrow QRS tachycardia of around 214/min. (2) Clearly visible P waves in V_2 (arrowheads). (3) **QRS alternans** which is best seen in V_4 (arrowheads). (4) When the ECG was in sinus rhythm, WPW pattern (preexcitation) was seen.

(12) ACCELERATED JUNCTIONAL RHYTHM

This arrhythmia is due to acceleration of the junctional pacemaker. The ECG shows normal QRS complexes at a rate of approximately 100/min (from 60-130/min). Since the junctional rate is faster than the sinus rate, the ventricles are depolarized by the junctional pacemaker and the atria by the sinoatrial node. Depolarization of the ventricles and the atria by 2 different pacemakers at different rates results in the phenomenon of **atrioventricular (AV) dissociation**. A sinus P wave, which occurs fortuitously at a time when the AV node is nonrefractory, will be conducted anterogradely to depolarize the ventricles, giving rise to a **capture beat** (Fig. 5.22).

Accelerated junctional rhythm is seen in acute myocardial infarction, digitalis intoxication, acute myocarditis and after the cardiac surgery. It is usually a transient arrhythmia and requires no specific treatment.

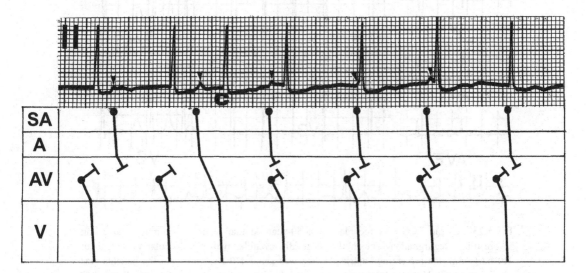

Fig. 5.22   Accelerated junctional rhythm. Note: (1) Accelerated junctional pacemaker rate of 83/min. (2) AV dissociation. (3) Sinus capture beat (C). Laddergram illustrates mechanism of AV dissociation and sinus capture.

(13) ATRIAL FIBRILLATION

Atrial fibrillation is the commonest sustained cardiac arrhythmia, with an increasing frequency in elderly people. It is also the most frequent cause of **"Irregular narrow QRS complex (<0.12 sec) tachycardia"**. The most common causes of atrial fibrillation are hypertension, heart failure, ischaemic heart disease, mitral valve disease, thyrotoxicosis and old age. The ECG in atrial fibrillation shows no P waves but instead **fibrillatory ("f") waves**, which result in an undulating baseline, are seen (Figs. 5.23 and 5.24). Atrial fibrillation is described as fine or coarse depending on the size of the "f" waves (Fig. 5.25). The ventricular rate in undigitalized patients is usually rapid and may vary between 140 to 180/min and the rhythm is very irregular. Verapamil or beta-blockers is used to reduce the ventricular rate in atrial fibrillation by decreasing conduction in the AV node. However, in some older patients where conduction in the AV node is already impaired, the ventricular rate may be normal and no treatment is necessary with regard to rate control.

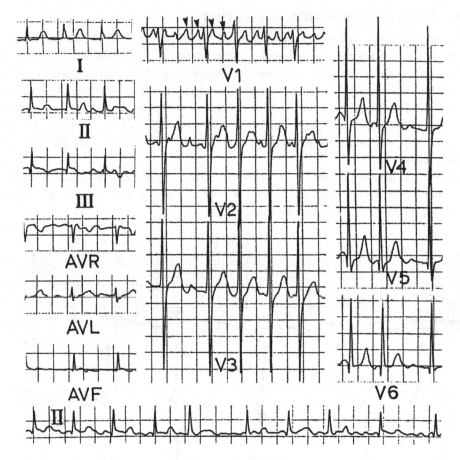

Fig. 5.23 12-lead ECG was recorded in a 50-year-old man with a flail mitral valve and severe mitral regurgitation. The rhythm is totally irregular with a ventricular rate of about 110 beats/min (the presenting ventricular rate was about 170 beats/min and the patients was given verapamil). No sinus P waves are seen and they are replaced by irregular fibrillatory "f" waves (arrowheads in V_1). The ECG is typical of atrial fibrillation.

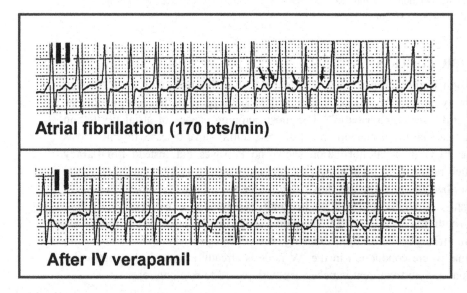

Atrial fibrillation (170 bts/min)

After IV verapamil

Fig. 5.24 The top panel shows **atrial fibrillation** (with a ventricular rate of about 170 beats/min) in a patient with mitral valve disease. The arrows indicate fibrillatory "f" waves. The bottom panel also shows atrial fibrillation, except that the ventricular rate is now much slower (about 105 beats/min) due to the cardio-depressant effect of verapamil on the AV node.

The following are the 2 most important issues in management: (1) rate versus rhythm control (i.e. accepting the atrial fibrillation but maintaining a slower heart rate by using drugs like verapamil and beta-blockers versus attempting to maintain sinus rhythm by either using anti-arrhythmic drugs like sotalol, propafenone or amiodarone or by catheter ablation (2) accessing the risk for thromboembolic stroke after which a decision is made whether the patient requires oral anticoagulant therapy or not.

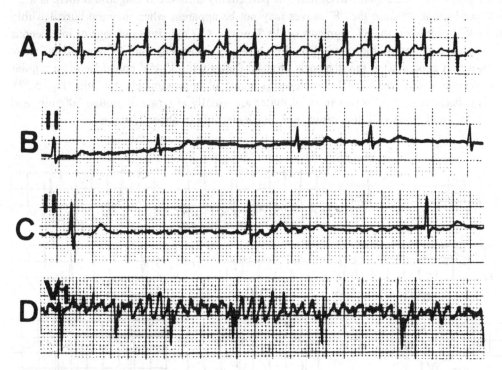

Fig. 5.25 Atrial fibrillation. Panel A is the ECG of a 36-year-old woman with rheumatic mitral stenosis. It shows atrial fibrillation with a very rapid ventricular rate. Panel B was recorded from the same patient after digitalization. The ventricular rate is now excessively slow, due to too much digoxin. Panel C, which was recorded from a 60-year-old man, shows atrial fibrillation with third degree (complete) AV block. The ventricular rate is very slow (31/min) and regular. Panel D is the ECG of a 26-year-old man with rheumatic mitral and aortic valve disease. The "f" waves are much bigger in amplitude compared to those in Panels A to C. This type of atrial fibrillation is termed "coarse atrial fibrillation" in contrast to the atrial fibrillation in panels B and C which can be described as "fine atrial fibrillation".

(14) ATRIAL FLUTTER

Atrial flutter is considerably less common than atrial fibrillation. The causes and management of atrial flutter and atrial fibrillation are similar. The ECG in atrial flutter is characteristic and is reflected by **"saw-tooth" flutter ("F") waves**. These are most apparent in leads II, III and aVF (Fig. 5.26). However, in lead V_1, discrete P waves are very often seen (Fig. 5.28). The ventricular rate, as well as the regularity of the rhythm, depends on the ratio of AV conduction. Atrial flutter is particularly difficult to diagnose if there is a 2:1 AV conduction, because the "F" waves may not be apparent when they are buried within the QRS complexes, the ST segments or the T waves. Carotid sinus massage or intravenous adenosine may reveal the concealed "F" waves by increasing the AV conduction ratio. However, a good clue to the diagnosis of atrial flutter with 2:1 AV conduction is a regular tachycardia with narrow QRS complexes at a rate of approximately 150/min (Fig. 5.27). This is because the "F" waves in atrial flutter are usually at a rate of around 300/min, and a 2:1 AV conduction will thus result in a ventricular rate of about 150/min.

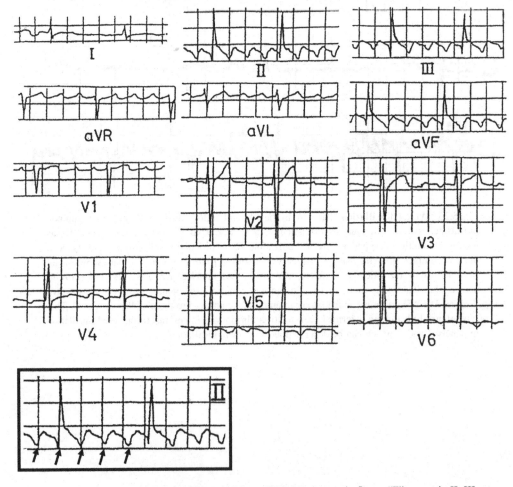

Fig. 5.26   Atrial flutter. Note: (1) Rapid (about 280/min) saw tooth, flutter "F" waves in II, III and aVF (arrows in the bottom box). (2) The ventricular rate is around 70/min due to a 4:1 AV conduction ratio.

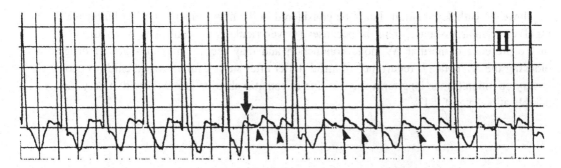

Fig. 5.27 Atrial flutter with 2:1 AV conduction ratio and a ventricular rate of 150/min. During 2:1 AV conduction, the flutter "F" waves are hidden as they are buried within the QRS complexes, ST segments or T waves. They are evident only when the AV conduction ratio is increased resulting in a slower ventricular rate (arrow). Arrowheads indicate flutter "F" waves (see text in page 94).

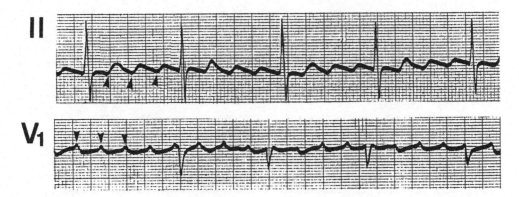

Fig. 5.28 Top panel, which was recorded in II, shows atrial flutter with a 4:1 AV conduction ratio. The flutter "F" waves are clearly seen and have a saw-tooth appearance (arrowheads). The rate of the "F" waves is unusually slow (214/min), because the patient was on an anti-arrhythmic drug. In the bottom panel, which was recorded in V_1, discrete P waves are seen (arrowheads) and the AV conduction ratio is variable.

In patients with atrial flutter who have been given an anti-arrhythmic drug, the rate of the "F" wave may be markedly reduced (Fig. 5.28). As in atrial fibrillation, verapamil or beta-blocker are the drugs of choice if the ventricular rate is rapid. However, atrial flutter is easily terminated by low energy electrical cardioversion, and this method of treatment is frequently employed if the arrhythmia requires to be terminated acutely. As with atrial fibrillation, accessing the risk for thromboembolic stroke is essential, after which a decision is made whether the patient requires oral anticoagulant therapy or not.

However, catheter ablation should be considered in the management of atrial flutter with rapid ventricular response. This is because: (1) ventricular rate control is often difficult in the presence of normal AV node conduction and may require high dosages of drugs blocking the AV node (2) recurrence of atrial flutter after successful electrical cardioversion is very common (3) the long term success rate of catheter ablation is > 90% with a very low complication rate of < 1%.

CHAPTER 6

VENTRICULAR ARRHYTHMIAS

Ventricular arrhythmias are common and frequently present a challenge as well as a dilemma to the clinician.

(1) VENTRICULAR ECTOPIC BEATS
(VENTRICULAR EXTRASYSTOLES, PREMATURE VENTRICULAR CONTRACTIONS)

Ventricular ectopic beats are commonly seen and they often present as palpitations. However, it is important to know that many people with frequent ventricular ectopic beats are asymptomatic. The ECG recognition of a ventricular ectopic beat depends on the following 2 criteria:

(1) It occurs prematurely
(2) The widened and bizarre-looking QRS complex is not preceded by a premature P wave

The **compensatory pause** is described as being "complete" when the interval between the 2 sinus beats flanking an ectopic beat is equal to 2 sinus cycles, and "incomplete" when it is shorter (Figs. 5.10, 6.1 and 6.2). A complete compensatory pause results when the sinoatrial node is not depolarized by an ectopic beat and the sinus cycle is not reset, whereas an incomplete compensatory pause is seen when the sinoatrial node is prematurely depolarized.

The main differential diagnosis of a ventricular ectopic beat is a supraventricular ectopic beat with **aberrant ventricular conduction** – a term used to describe a supraventricular beat which is conducted to only 1 ventricle because of transient bundle branch block. This phenomenon occurs because the refractory periods of the 2 bundle branches are frequently unequal. The right bundle branch usually has a longer refractory period compared to the left.

A late supraventricular beat will be conducted through both bundle branches because they will have fully recovered from the previous depolarization. A very early supraventricular beat will find both bundle branches refractory and the impulse will be blocked. A supraventricular beat of intermediate prematurity may find 1 bundle branch (usually the right bundle branch) still refractory, while the other has recovered fully. This beat will be conducted through the recovered branch, giving rise to a ventricular complex with a bundle branch block pattern. This phenomenon is termed "aberrant ventricular conduction". Although the QRS complex is widened in a supraventricular ectopic beat with aberrant ventricular conduction, it is less bizarre looking than a ventricular ectopic beat, being frequently similar to a bundle branch block morphology – right more common than left (Fig. 6.3). A longer preceding R–R interval increases the refractory period of the bundle branches, thus favouring aberrant ventricular conduction for the same degree of prematurity. This phenomenon is termed the **"Ashman's phenomenon"** (Fig. 6.4).

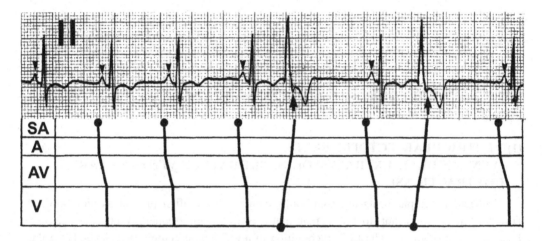

Fig. 6.1 This ECG is the second panel of Fig. 6.5. It shows frequent **uniform ventricular ectopic beats**. Arrows indicate P waves which have resulted from retrograde depolarization of the atria. Arrowheads indicate sinus P waves. Note that the compensatory pause is incomplete. This is because the ventricular ectopic beats are conducted retrogradely through the AV node and across the atria to the sinoatrial node which is prematurely depolarized. This results in a resetting of the sinus cycle.

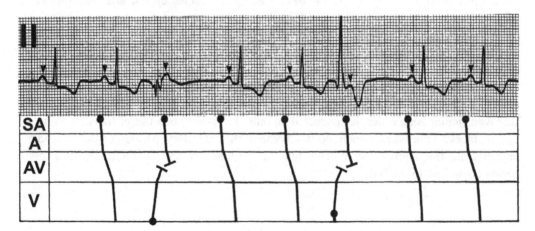

Fig. 6.2 This ECG is the third panel of Fig. 6.5. Note: (1) **Multiform ventricular ectopic beats**. (2) AV dissociation. (3) Complete compensatory pause.

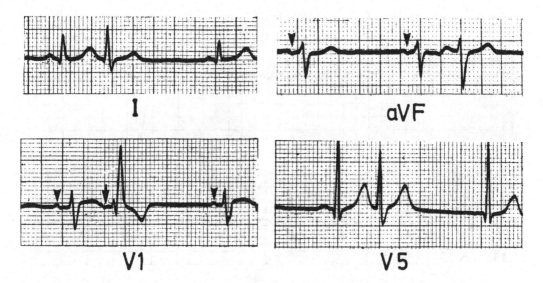

Fig. 6.3 Atrial ectopic beats with aberrant ventricular conduction. Arrow indicates atrial ectopic beat and arrowheads, sinus P waves. Note: (1) Ventricular complex following each atrial ectopic beat has a right bundle branch block morphology. (2) Incomplete compensatory pause.

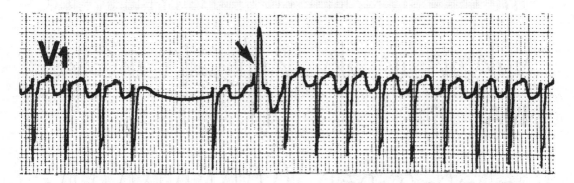

Fig. 6.4 Ashman's phenomenon. ECG shows a run of supraventricular tachycardia which terminates spontaneously for a brief period before it is resumed. The ventricular complex labelled with an arrow shows a right bundle branch block morphology due to aberrant ventricular conduction, although it is not earlier than all the other ventricular complexes which are normally conducted. This is because it is preceded by a longer R–R interval. This phenomenon is known as the "Ashman's phenomenon".

Figure 6.5 shows the **Lown's grading system** for ventricular ectopic beats.

The grading is as follows: Grade 0 – none; Grade 1 – occasional (< 30/hour); Grade 2 – frequent (≥ 30/hour); Grade 3 – multiform; Grade 4A – 2 consecutive ventricular ectopic beats (couplets); Grade 4B – 3 or more consecutive ventricular ectopic beats; Grade 5 – "R on T".

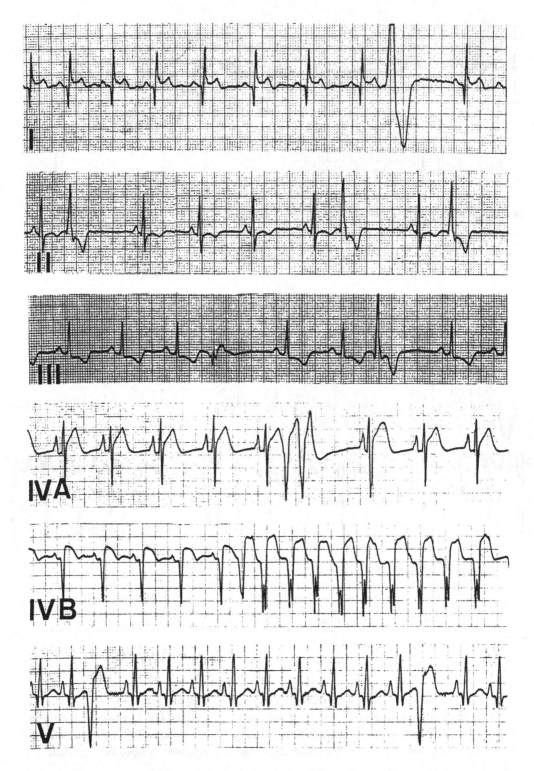

Fig. 6.5 Lown's grading system of ventricular ectopic beats. Grade 1 = uniform and infrequent (< 30/hr). Grade 2 = uniform and frequent (30 or >/hr). Grade 3 = multiform. Grade 4A = 2 consecutive beats (pairs or couplets). Grade 4B = 3 or more consecutive beats. Grade 5 = "R on T".

Uniform ventricular ectopic beats have the same **coupling interval** (i.e. the interval between the ectopic beat and the preceding sinus beat) and morphology. Multiform ventricular ectopic beats very frequently have different coupling intervals and morphologies, indicating that they arise from different foci. **"R on T"** ventricular ectopic beats occur very prematurely at the apices or the downslope of the T waves of the preceding sinus beats. In the past, it was strongly believed that if they occur in acute myocardial infarction, the risk of ventricular fibrillation is greatly increased. However, currently, there is uncertainty whether this increased risk of ventricular fibrillation is seen in all "R on T" ventricular ectopic beats.

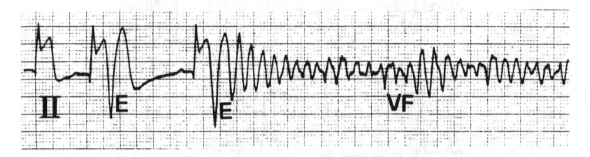

Fig. 6.6 **"R on T" ventricular ectopic beats** (E) precipitating ventricular fibrillation (VF) in a patient with inferior STEMI.

The first ventricular ectopic beat sometimes starts a run of **ventricular bigeminy**. This is because the compensatory pause which follows results in a longer R–R interval preceding the next sinus beat, and this encourages the emergence of another ventricular ectopic beat. This phenomenon is called the **"rule of bigeminy"** which is seen in both ventricular as well as supraventricular ectopic beats. Figure 6.7 shows a case of ventricular bigeminy.

Ventricular ectopic beats are **ubiquitous** and are commonly seen in normal people as well as in those with various structural heart disease such as acute and chronic myocardial infarction, hypertension with left ventricular hypertrophy, cardiomyopathy, and valvular heart disease.

Lown's grading system was at first used as a **prognostic classification** – the higher the grade, the worse the prognosis. However, over the years, it became clear that this pertains mainly to patients with **acute myocardial infarction and ischaemia**. In other situations, prognosis is related not just to the complexity or grading of the ventricular ectopic beats, but more importantly as to whether there is any structural heart disease and to the degree of any left ventricular dysfunction.

With regard to **prognosis**, in an individual with frequent ventricular ectopic beats, but who has a normal left ventricular function and no structural heart disease, the prognosis is usually highly favorable. These ventricular ectopic beats frequently arise from the outflow tract of the right ventricle and has a left bundle branch block with an inferior axis morphology (Fig. 6.7). No treatment is needed if there are no symptoms. However, if the individual is significantly distressed by palpitations, a beta-blocker and if necessary an antiarrhythmic drug can be given to suppress the ectopy.

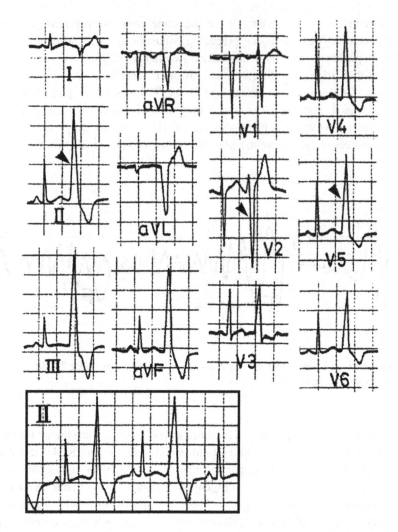

Fig. 6.7 Ventricular bigeminy. Note that a ventricular ectopic beat (arrowheads in V_2, V_5 and II) follows every sinus beat resulting in ventricular bigeminy. The ventricular ectopic beats have a left bundle branch block morphology, indicating that they have arisen from the right ventricle.

In an opposite situation, a patient with a significantly impaired left ventricular function (e.g. left ventricular ejection fraction < 30%) due to chronic myocardial infarction or some other structural heart disease, which is associated with frequent ventricular ectopic beats will have an increase risk of ventricular fibrillation. These patients need to be considered for implantation of an implantable cardioverter-defibrillator.

(2) DIGITALIS INTOXICATION

The **"digitalis effect"** refers to the ECG changes that are typically seen in patients taking digitalis. It consists of the downward scooping of the ST-T complex and does not imply digitalis intoxication (Fig. 6.8).

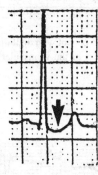

Fig. 6.8 "Digitalis effect". Lead II in a patient who was prescribed digoxin. Note the downward scooping of the ST-T complex (arrow).

The following arrhythmias occurring either alone, or especially in combination, are highly suggestive of **digitalis intoxication**: (1) Unifocal but multiform ventricular ectopic beats (Fig. 6.9) – these ventricular ectopic beats have identical coupling intervals but different morphologies, implying that they may have arisen from the same focus but have different exits arising from the same reentrant circuit. (2) Mobitz type I second degree (Wenckebach phenomenon) and third degree AV block with narrow QRS complexes (3) Accelerated junctional rhythm (4) Sinoatrial block (5) **Bidirectional ventricular tachycardia**. This is a very rare arrhythmia. The ECG shows alternation in the polarity of the ventricular complexes (Fig. 6.10). In a patient who is on digoxin and presents with bidirectional ventricular tachycardia, digitalis intoxication is very likely. The risk of digitalis intoxication is significantly increased in hypokalaemia.

Certain arrhythmias such as right or left bundle branch block, Mobitz type II second degree AV block and complete heart block (with wide QRS complexes) are very rare in digitalis intoxication.

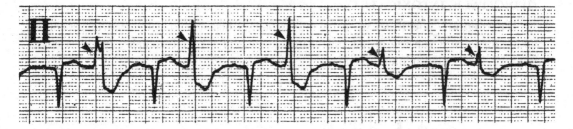

Fig. 6.9 Unifocal, multiform ventricular ectopic beats in a patient with digitalis intoxication. Note the constant coupling interval but varying morphologies of the ventricular ectopic beats (arrowheads).

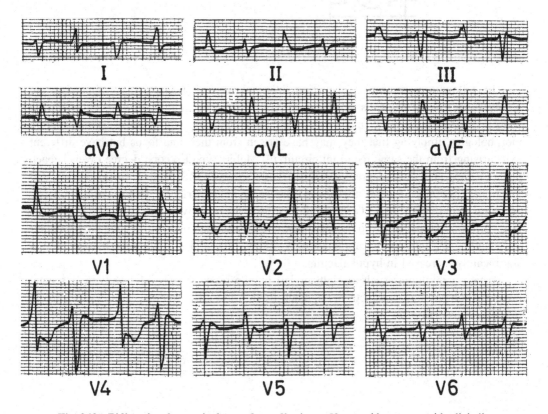

Fig. 6.10 Bidirectional ventricular tachycardia in a 58-year-old woman with digitalis intoxication. Note that the polarity of the consecutive QRS complexes is alternately positive and negative in all the leads except for V_1 and V_2.

(3) MONOMORPHIC VENTRICULAR TACHYCARDIA (see Epilogue page 116)

Monomorphic ventricular tachycardia is defined as 3 or more consecutive ventricular ectopic beats at a rate of ≥ 100/min (4B in Lown's grading of ventricular ectopic beats). It is described as sustained when it lasts longer than 30 sec or if it requires electrical cardioversion for haemodynamic instability and nonsustained when it is shorter.

The 12-lead ECG in ventricular tachycardia shows wide (≥ 0.12 sec) and bizarre looking QRS complexes frequently at a rapid rate of between 140 to 200/min (Figs. 6.11-6.13). The ECG differentiation between ventricular tachycardia and supraventricular tachycardia with aberrant ventricular conduction requires experience and skill.

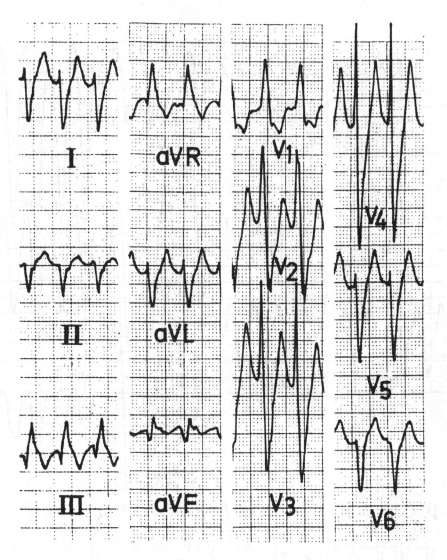

Fig. 6.11 Ventricular tachycardia. Note: (1) Rapid ventricular rate of 158/min. (2) Regular and wide (0.16 sec) QRS complexes. (3) Monophasic R wave in V_1. (4) rS complex in V_5 and V_6. (5) Axis of approximately +180°.

The points in favour of ventricular tachycardia vs supraventricular tachycardia with aberrant ventricular conduction are as follows:

(1) Atrioventricular (AV) dissociation (Figs. 6.15 and 6.26)
(2) Capture beats with narrow QRS morphology, in the midst of rapid and wide ventricular complexes
(3) Fusion beats (Fig. 6.13)
(4) "Concordant pattern" which means that the polarity of all the QRS complexes in the praecordial leads is either negative or positive (Fig. 6.12)
(5) An indeterminate QRS axis (Fig. 6.16)

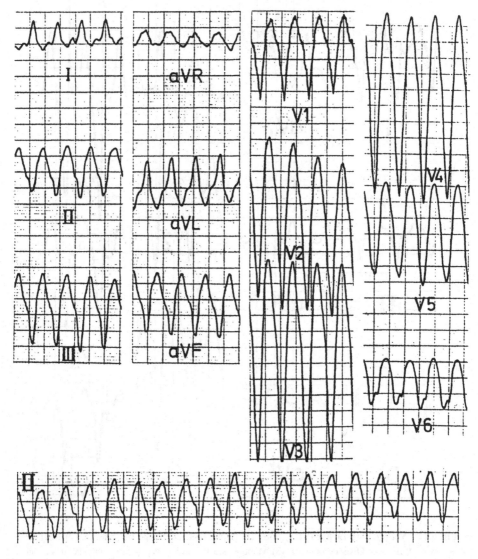

Fig. 6.12 Ventricular tachycardia showing the negative concordance pattern. Note: (1) Regular, wide QRS tachycardia (190/min). (2) All the QRS complexes in the praecordial leads from V_1 to V_6 are negative in polarity.

On the other hand, the ECG in supraventricular tachycardia with aberrant ventricular conduction very frequently show a 1:1 P-QRS relationship (i.e. one P wave to every QRS complex) and widened QRS complexes with a typical bundle branch block morphology – right more common than left (Fig. 6.14).

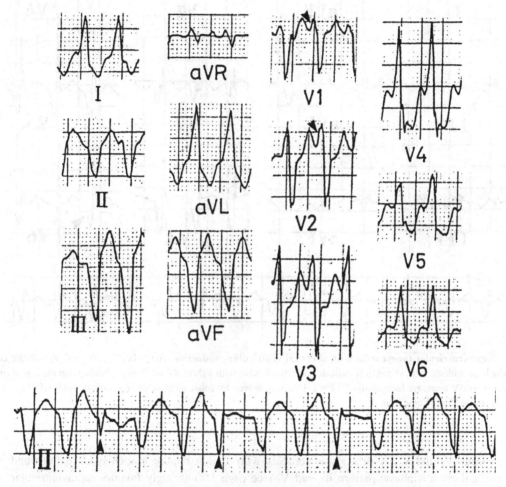

Fig. 6.13 Ventricular tachycardia in a patient with acute myocardial infarction. Note: (1) Regular, wide QRS tachycardia of around 166/min. (2) The QRS morphology superficially resembles a left bundle branch pattern, except that the r waves in V_1 and V_2 (arrowheads) are broad thus favouring ventricular ectopy. (3) The rhythm strip in the lower part of the ECG shows fusion beats (arrowheads) which are of different morphologies.

Unfortunately, AV dissociation (which is almost diagnostic of ventricular tachycardia) is present in about 50% but is visible in about only 25% of ventricular tachycardia cases. Capture beats, fusion beats, a concordant pattern (especially negative concordance) and an indeterminate axis, although all highly specific for ventricular tachycardia, are all only occasionally present. Because of this, there has been much emphasis in recent years on the analysis of the morphology of the ventricular complexes in the 12-lead ECG, especially

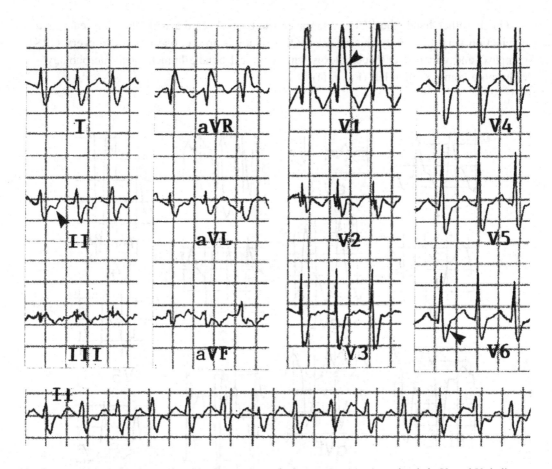

Fig. 6.14   Supraventricular tachycardia with aberrant ventricular conduction. Arrowheads in V_1 and V_6 indicate complete right bundle branch block. Arrowhead in II indicates inverted P wave with a short RP interval suggesting that the supraventricular tachycardia is an AV reentrant tachycardia (WPW). This was proven by subsequent electrophysiology study. (ECG courtesy of Assistant Professor Pipin Kojodjojo).

in leads V_1 and V_6. A ventricular complex with a right bundle branch block pattern and particularly a triphasic pattern in lead V_1 (see page 118) strongly favours supraventricular tachycardia with aberrant ventricular conduction (Fig. 6.14 and Fig. 6.16). On the other hand, both a monophasic R wave or a diphasic qR complex in lead V_1 and a rS or QS complex in lead V_6, strongly favour the diagnosis of ventricular tachycardia (Fig. 6.11). When the QRS complexes show a left bundle branch block pattern, both ventricular tachycardia and a supraventricular tachycardia with aberrant ventricular conduction (presenting with the less common manifestation of a left bundle branch block) have to be considered. In leads V_1/V_2, a wide r wave (≥ 0.04 sec) and a slow S wave descent which is notched or slurred with an interval of ≥ 0.06 sec between the beginning of the QRS complex and the nadir of the S wave and also a qR pattern in lead V_6 all strongly favour the diagnosis of ventricular tachycardia (Fig. 6.13). On the other hand, a narrow r wave and a rapid S wave descent in V_1/V_2 favours left bundle branch block aberrancy (Fig. 7.6).

Sustained ventricular tachycardia is usually associated with coronary artery, myocardial or other structural heart disease. It is a serious condition since it may deteriorate to ventricular fibrillation. Intravenous amiodarone is the drug of choice. If there is no response to pharmacological therapy or if the patient presents with hypotension, electrical cardioversion is necessary (Fig. 6.17).

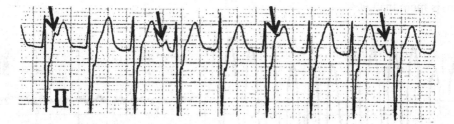

Fig. 6.15 Atrioventricular dissociation in a patient with ventricular tachycardia. Arrows indicate sinus P waves which are buried in a run of regular wide QRS complex tachycardia reflecting ventricular tachycardia.

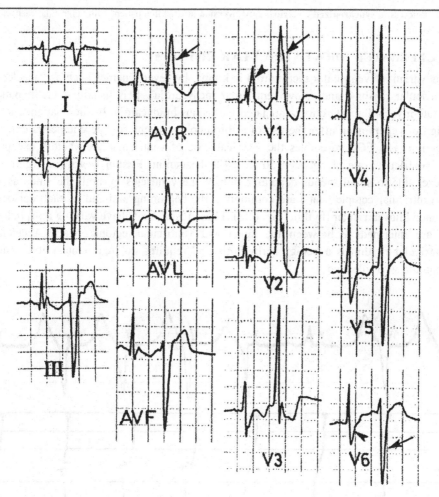

Fig. 6.16 The first beat in each lead shows sinus rhythm with complete right bundle branch block conduction (arrowheads in V_1 and V_6) which is a typical feature of aberrant ventricular conduction. The second beat is a ventricular ectopic beat (arrows in V_1, V_6 and AVR) which shows the typical features of ventricular ectopy – dominant R wave and S wave in V_1 and V_6 respectively, as well as an indeterminate QRS axis of about −120°.

(4) CLINICAL PERSPECTIVE

Despite difficulties in differentiating between ventricular tachycardia and supraventricular tachycardia with aberrant ventricular conduction, it is important to know that in unselected patients presenting with regular wide QRS complex tachycardia, up to 80% of the cases will turn out to be ventricular tachycardia and in patients with prior myocardial infarction, the figure is more than 90%.

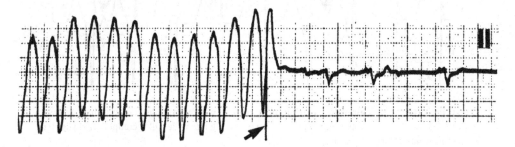

Fig. 6.17   Successful **synchronized electrical cardioversion** (arrow) in a patient with ventricular tachycardia.

(5) ACCELERATED IDIOVENTRICULAR RHYTHM

This variant of ventricular tachycardia is known by several names such as "accelerated idioventricular rhythm" and "slow ventricular tachycardia". It is usually seen in patients with acute myocardial infarction associated with sinus bradycardia. In such patients, it may be a sign of **reperfusion** after the use of a thrombolytic agent or a percutaneous coronary intervention. The ECG resembles the classical type of ventricular tachycardia except for a slow ventricular rate of between 50 to < 100 beats/min. **Fusion beats** (i.e. ventricular complexes due to simultaneous depolarization of the ventricles by both the sinus as well as the ventricular ectopic beats) are common at the beginning and end of each episode of accelerated idioventricular rhythm (Fig. 6.18). These fusion beats have varying morphologies which are intermediate between the sinus and ventricular ectopic beats. Accelerated idioventricular rhythm is a benign arrhythmia and requires no treatment as it is usually transient and well tolerated.

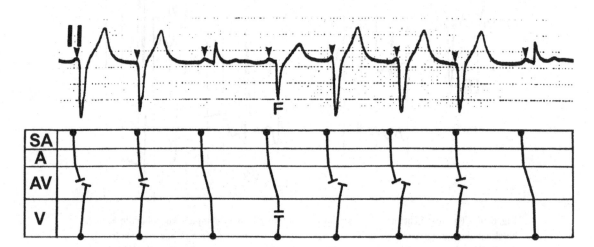

Fig. 6.18   Accelerated idioventricular rhythm. Note: (1) Termination and onset of accelerated idioventricular rhythm. (2) AV dissociation. (F = fusion beat). Arrowheads indicate sinus P waves.

(6) POLYMORPHIC VENTRICULAR TACHYCARDIA and TORSADES DE POINTES

Unlike monomorphic ventricular tachycardia where the morphology of all the QRS complexes are similar in a particular lead, in polymorphic ventricular tachycardia, there is a continuous variation in morphology and polarity of the QRS complexes. An important clinical subclassification of polymorphic ventricular tachycardia is between those where the QTc interval is normal (Fig. 6.19) and those where it is prolonged (Fig. 6.20). The latter category is called "torsades de pointes" which is a French term. In the classical form of torsades de pointes, there is twisting and turning of the QRS complexes around the isoelectric line, resulting in their apices being positive and negative for a few beats at a time (Fig. 6.21).

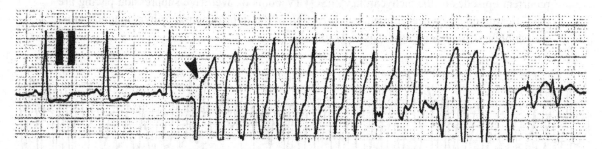

Fig. 6.19 Polymorphic ventricular tachycardia (arrowhead) with a normal QTc interval.

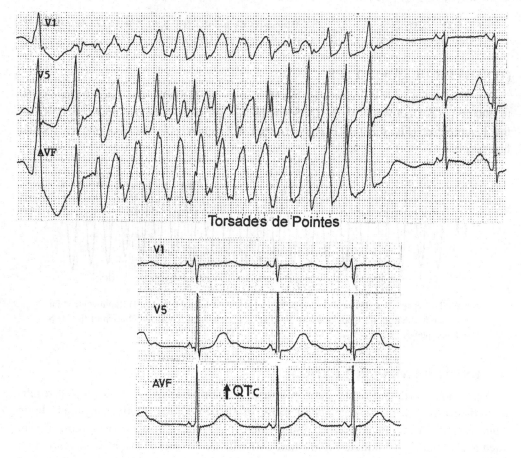

Fig. 6.20 Top panel shows **torsades de pointes**. Bottom panel shows sinus rhythm with a markedly prolonged QTc interval of 0.64 second.

111

In polymorphic ventricular tachycardia where the QTc interval is normal, the most common cause is acute myocardial infarction or ischaemic heart disease and the major complication is ventricular fibrillation. If the tachycardia is sustained, electrical cardioversion should be performed. IV amiodarone should be given for recurrent short runs of tachycardia. Polymorphic ventricular tachycardia with normal QTc interval is also seen in Brugada Syndrome (see page 114). In torsades de pointes, the prolonged QTc interval may be due to specific drugs like anti-arrhythmic drugs, hypokalaemia and hypomagnesaemia or hereditary long QT syndrome. The major complication of torsades de pointes is ventricular fibrillation. If the tachycardia is sustained, electrical cardioversion should be performed. For recurrent episodes of the tachycardia, MgSO4 IV bolus or overdrive suppression pacing are the 2 treatments of choice. Immediate correction of the hypokalaemia or hypomagnesaemia and stopping QT prolonging drugs is essential.

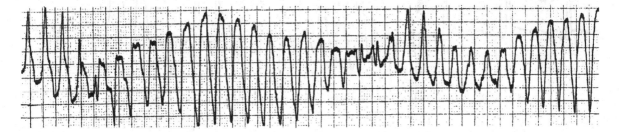

Fig. 6.21   ECG shows classical form of **torsades de pointes** (see text). The ECG when the patient was in sinus rhythm showed a markedly prolonged QTc interval.

(7) VENTRICULAR FLUTTER

Ventricular flutter is characterized by: (1) A very rapid ventricular rate of around 260 to 300/min; (2) Undulation of the QRS complexes; (3) No differentiation of the QRS or the T complexes (Fig. 6.22). If left uncorrected, it frequently degenerates into ventricular fibrillation.

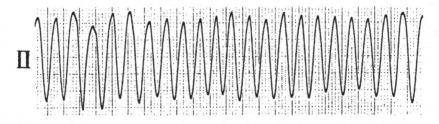

Fig. 6.22   Ventricular flutter in a terminally ill patient with stroke. Note: (1) Rapid ventricular rate of about 286/min. (2) Undulation of the QRS complexes. (3) No differentiation of the QRS and T complexes.

(8) VENTRICULAR FIBRILLATION

Ventricular fibrillation is the most serious of all cardiac arrhythmias because it results in cardiac arrest. It is the commonest cause of sudden cardiac death. Irreparable brain damage results if cardiopulmonary resuscitation or termination of the arrhythmia is not attempted within 3 to 4 minutes. Immediate defibrillation is crucial. The ECG in ventricular fibrillation shows completely irregular and chaotic deflections of varying amplitude and shape (Fig. 6.23).

Survivors of cardiac arrest are at a very high risk of having another episode of ventricular fibrillation. In the absence of a reversible cause for the initial episode of ventricular fibrillation, there is a very strong indication for an implantable cardioverter-defibrillator, which has been shown to improve survival.

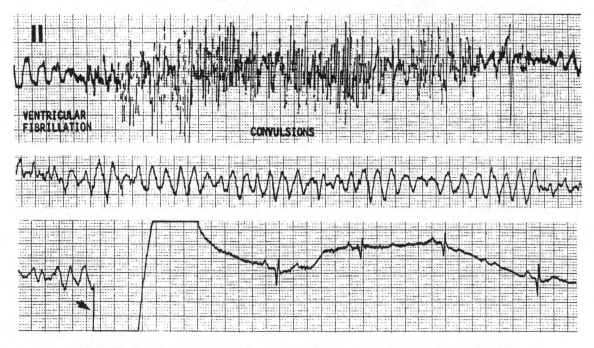

Fig. 6.23 **Ventricular fibrillation** in a patient with acute myocardial infarction. All 3 panels are continuous. After non-synchronized electrical cardioversion (arrow in bottom panel), sinus rhythm was restored.

(9) IDIOVENTRICULAR RHYTHM AND VENTRICULAR ASYSTOLE

In idioventricular rhythm, there is an extreme bradycardia with very wide and bizzare looking QRS complexes and absence of P waves. In ventricular asystole, only a straight line is seen (Fig. 6.24). Both these arrhythmias usually represent the final expression of a dying heart and resuscitative measures are often unsuccessful.

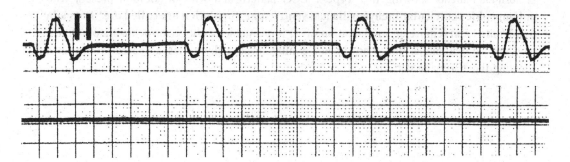

Fig. 6.24 **Idioventricular rhythm and ventricular asystole**. Top panel shows idioventricular rhythm. Note: (1) Absence of P waves. (2) Very wide and bizarre looking QRS complexes with an extremely slow ventricular rate (36/min). Bottom panel shows a straight line reflecting ventricular asystole.

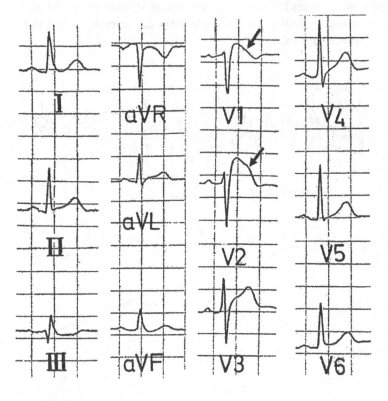

Fig. 6.25 Type 1 Brugada pattern. The J point is elevated ≥ 2 mm in V_1 and V_2. The elevated ST segment is coved shape (arrows in V_1 and V_2) and downsloping terminating in an inverted T wave.

(10) BRUGADA SYNDROME

The Brugada Syndrome is an inherited sodium ion channelopathy which is seen mainly in young males with structurally normal hearts. It is common in certain parts of South East Asia, especially in North East Thailand. The main clinical presentation is polymorphic ventricular tachycardia and ventricular fibrillation which occurs mainly at night. The ECG shows an elevated J point ≥ 2 mm in at least 2 of the following three leads – V_1, V_2, V_3 (most commonly V_1 and V_2). The elevated ST segment is coved shape and downsloping (looks like a sharkfin) terminating in an inverted T wave (Fig. 6.25). The QTc interval is normal. Patients showing this Type 1 ECG pattern and who in addition present with **polymorphic ventricular tachycardia** and **ventricular fibrillation are called the "Brugada Syndrome"** and require an implantation of an implantable cardioverter-defibrillator. Others who are asymptomatic, and who do not exhibit these arrhythmias are described as just showing the "Brugada Pattern".

EPILOGUE

(11) FASICULAR VENTRICULAR TACHYCARDIA

This uncommon form of ventricular tachycardia arises from the fascicles of the left bundle branch (posterior more frequently than anterior). It is usually seen in young males with structurally normal hearts. The ECG shows tachycardia with a relatively narrow right bundle branch block pattern (QRS duration from 0.11 to 0.14 second). Because of this, a wrong diagnosis of supraventricular tachycardia with aberrant ventricular conduction is frequently made. There is usually left axis deviation indicating that the ventricular tachycardia has arisen from the posterior fascicle. Like the other types of ventricular tachycardia, the amplitude of the S wave in V_6 is greater than that of the R wave, A-V dissociation, and much less commonly, capture and fusion beats are all seen. The unique feature about fasicular ventricular tachycardia is that it responds very well to verapamil compared to the other antiarrhythmic drugs and verapamil therefore is the drug of choice. Importantly, IV verapamil is contraindicated in most of the conventional types of ventricular tachycardia as it may cause marked haemodynamic deterioration and ventricular fibrillation.

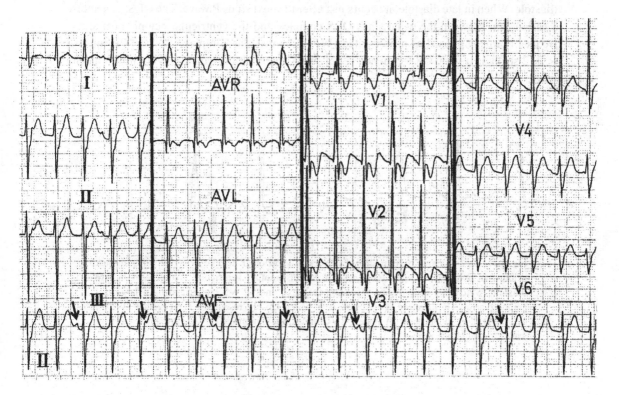

Fig. 6.26 12-lead ECG of a 26-year-old male with no structural heart disease, showing **Fasicular Ventricular Tachycardia**. Note: (1) Regular tachycardia (133/min) (2) Relatively narrow (> 0.10 sec) rSR′, right bundle branch block pattern ventricular complex in V_1 (3) S wave > R wave in V_6 (4) A-V dissociation in long lead II rhythm strip. Arrows indicate sinus P waves.

115

(12) "REGULAR WIDE QRS COMPLEX TACHYCARDIA" (see page 105)

The 3 main causes of "Regular wide QRS complex (≥ 0.12 sec) tachycardia" in order of frequency are (1) **Ventricular Tachycardia** (2) **Supraventricular Tachycardia with aberrant ventricular conduction** and occasionally (3) **AV reentrant antidromic tachycardia**. In the section on Preexcitation and Wolff-Parkinson-White Syndrome (see page 88), it was stated that the commonest arrhythmia in this condition is an AV reentrant **orthodromic** tachycardia where the cardiac impulse travels anterogradely down the AV node and retrogradely up the accessory pathway. The ECG here shows a regular narrow QRS complex (< 0.12 sec) tachycardia; AV reentrant **antidromic** tachycardia where the impulse travels anterogradely down the accessory pathway and retrogradely up the AV node is much less common. The ECG here shows regular wide QRS complex tachycardia simulating very closely ventricular tachycardia. How to differentiate between these 2 arrhythmias is beyond the scope of this book.

IV Amiodarone is generally effective for ventricular tachycardia, supraventricular tachycardia with aberrant ventricular conduction and AV reentrant antidromic tachycardia.

(13) VENTRICULAR ECTOPIC BEATS IN LATE DIASTOLE

A ventricular ectopic beat can occur very early ("R on T"), in the middle of, or in **late diastole**. When in late diastole, it occurs just after the next sinus P wave. The QRS is therefore a fusion beat between the usual sinus QRS complex and the ventricular ectopic beat and is frequently misdiagnosed as a preexcited (WPW) ventricular complex – a short PR interval (< 0.12 sec) and a wide QRS complex (≥ 0.12 sec), the beginning of which resembles a delta wave.

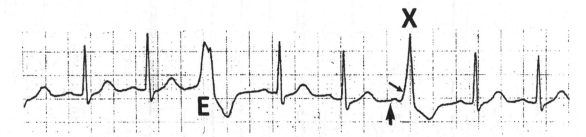

Fig. 6.27 In the above rhythm strip, E reflects a ventricular ectopic beat which begins just before the next sinus P wave (not seen). X reflects another ventricular ectopic beat in **late diastole**, which this time begins just after the next sinus P wave indicated by a large up-pointing arrow. X therefore is a fusion beat which closely resembles a preexcited (WPW) beat – (1) short PR interval (2) Wide QRS complex, the beginning of which resembles a delta wave (small oblique arrow).

CHAPTER 7

BUNDLE BRANCH BLOCK, HEMIBLOCK AND ATRIOVENTRICULAR (AV) BLOCK

The conducting system of the heart comprises the AV node and the bundle of His which divides into a right and a left bundle branch. The right bundle branch is a discrete structure from its origin to its termination, but the left bundle branch quickly divides into an anterior (superior) and a posterior (inferior) fascicle (Fig. 7.1). The infra-Hisian portion of the conducting system is therefore essentially trifascicular, consisting of the right bundle branch and the anterior and posterior fascicles of the left bundle branch.

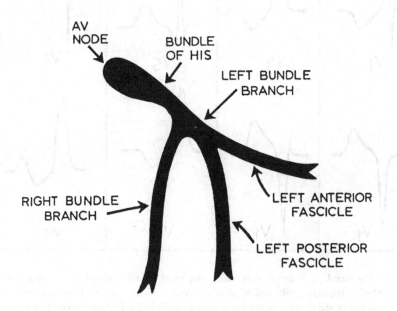

Fig. 7.1 Diagram illustrating the conducting system of the heart.

Block in conduction may be at the level of either the AV node, bundle of His, right or left bundle branch or the 2 fascicles of the left bundle branch, occurring singly or in different combinations. An isolated lesion of either the anterior or posterior fascicle of the left bundle branch is termed a hemiblock. The combination of right bundle branch block and either left anterior or posterior hemiblock is termed **bifascicular block**, because 2 of the 3 fascicles of the conducting system are involved.

(1) BUNDLE BRANCH BLOCK

The ECG in **right bundle branch block** shows: (1) A widened QRS complex (due to a wide R' wave) with either a **triphasic** (rSR') or an M (RsR') shaped pattern and secondary T wave inversion in leads V_1 to V_3. (2) A wide and slurred S wave in leads V_5, V_6, I and aVL (Figs. 7.2 and 7.3). The right bundle branch block is described as being **complete** if the width of the QRS complex is ≥ 0.12 sec, and **incomplete** if it is < 0.12 sec. The axis in isolated right bundle branch block is normal. An axis ≥ −45° or ≥ +120° indicates co-existing left anterior or left posterior hemiblock respectively (Figs. 7.5 and 2.17).

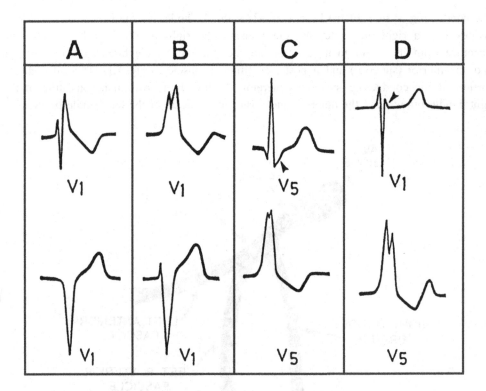

Fig. 7.2 Top panel. A, B and C show morphologies of the QRS complexes in **right bundle branch block** – triphasic (rSR') and M (RsR') pattern in V_1 are seen in A and B respectively. C shows widening and slurring of the S wave (arrowhead) in V_5. D shows **normal variant rSr' pattern** in V_1. Arrowhead indicates r' wave (see text in page 119). **Bottom panel.** A, B, C and D show morphologies of the QRS complexes in **left bundle branch block** – monophasic (QS) and rS ventricular complexes in V_1 are seen in A and B respectively. Widened and slightly notched R wave and M shaped R wave in V_5 are seen in C and D respectively.

Right bundle branch block is seen in atrial septal defect (about 90% of cases and usually the incomplete variety), acute myocardial infarction, ischaemic and hypertensive heart disease, acute pulmonary embolus, degenerative disease of the conducting system and after operation for tetralogy of Fallot and ventricular septal defect. Complete right bundle branch block also occurs in approximately 0.2% and incomplete bundle branch block in about 3% of the general population.

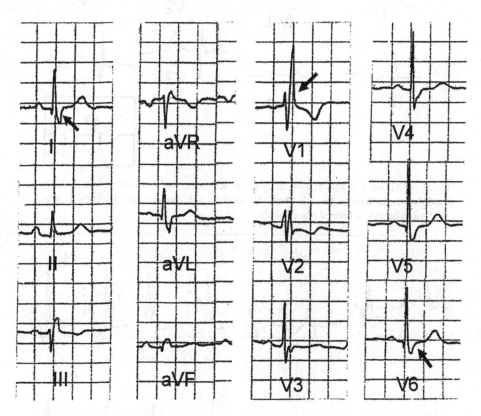

Fig. 7.3 Complete right bundle branch block in an 80-year-old woman with hypertension. Note: (1) rSR′ in V$_1$ (arrow). The QRS complex is widened (0.14 sec). (2) Slurring and widening of the S wave in V$_5$, V$_6$, I and aVL (arrows in V$_6$ and I). The axis is normal (about +15°).

A **rSr′ pattern** with a narrow QRS duration of ≤ 0.10 sec and a very small (≤ 1-2 mm) terminal r′ wave is commonly seen in leads V$_1$ or V$_1$ and V$_2$ (Fig. 7.2). This **normal variant** should not be overread and wrongly diagnosed as incomplete right bundle branch block. (Goldberger AL, Goldberger ZD, Shvilkin A. Goldberger's Clinical Electrocardiography. A simplified approach. Elsevier Saunders. Philadelphia, PA. 2013: 57).

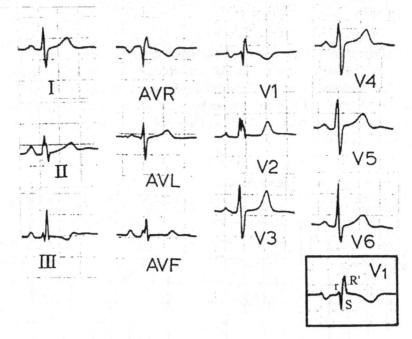

Fig. 7.4 ECG from a patient with an ostium secundum atrial septal defect showing an **incomplete right bundle branch block**. V_1 shows a rSR' pattern and the QRS duration is < 0.12 sec. The axis is normal (about +60°).

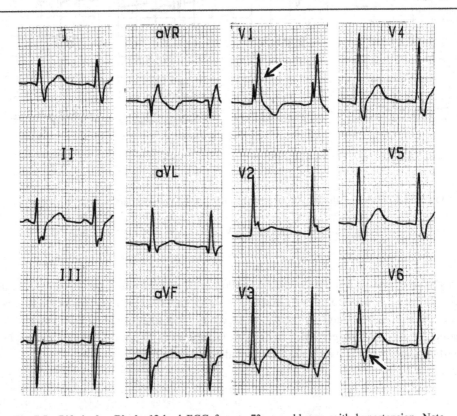

Fig. 7.5 Bifasicular Block. 12-lead ECG from a 73-year-old man with hypertension. Note (1) Complete right bundle branch block (arrows in V_1 and V_6 [QRS > 0.12 sec]). (2) The axis is −50° indicating coexisting left anterior hemiblock. See Fig. 2.17 for complete right bundle branch block and left posterior hemiblock.

In **left bundle branch block**, the widened ventricular complexes are usually monophasic and slightly notched or slurred in leads V_5 and V_6. Less commonly, they are M shaped. There is also secondary ST segment depression and T wave inversion and an absence of q waves in these 2 leads. The right praecordial leads (i.e. leads V_1 and V_2) usually show deep Q waves and less commonly, rS complexes. ST segment elevation simulating anterior STEMI is very frequently seen (Fig. 7.6). As with right-bundle branch block, left bundle branch block may either be complete (≥ 0.12 sec) or incomplete (< 0.12 sec). Left bundle branch block seldom occur in normal people. The common causes are acute myocardial infarction, ischaemic and hypertensive heart disease, dilated cardiomyopathy and degenerative disease of the conducting system.

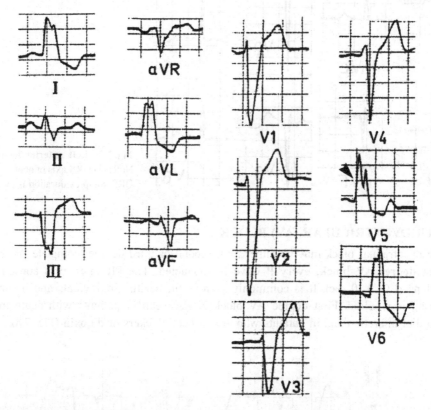

Fig. 7.6 Complete left bundle branch block in a 67-year-old woman. Note: (1) Wide (0.16 sec) M shaped QRS complex, with an absence of a q wave in V_5 (arrowhead) and notching of the R wave in V_6. Secondary ST depression and T wave inversion in V_5 and V_6. (2) rS complex and ST elevation in V_1-V_4.

(2) HEMIBLOCK

Left anterior hemiblock is diagnosed when the axis is $\geq -45°$. The width of the QRS complex is either normal or minimally widened (Fig. 7.7). **Left posterior hemiblock** is considerably less common than left anterior hemiblock and it is also more difficult to diagnose with confidence. The diagnosis can be made if the axis is $> +120°$, but a vertical heart, right ventricular hypertrophy and chronic obstructive lung disease must first be excluded. The causes of hemiblock and bundle branch block are generally similar.

If the ECG shows a combination of complete right bundle branch block with either a left anterior (Fig. 7.5) or less commonly a left posterior (Fig. 2.17) hemiblock, it is termed a **bifasicular block**.

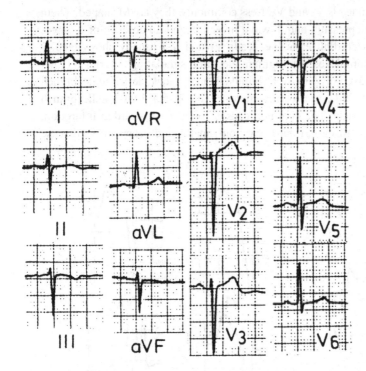

Fig. 7.7 **Left anterior hemiblock**. Note: (1) QRS axis of about −60° (2) QRS complex duration is normal.

(3) ATRIOVENTRICULAR (AV) BLOCK

Atrioventricular block may be either first, second or third degree (complete AV block). In **first degree AV block**, every P wave is conducted. The PR interval is constant and is prolonged (> 0.20 sec). It is commonly seen in fit, healthy individuals and no specific treatment is required. First degree AV block is also seen in patients with acute inferior myocardial infarction and in patients who are on beta-blockers or digoxin (Fig. 7.8).

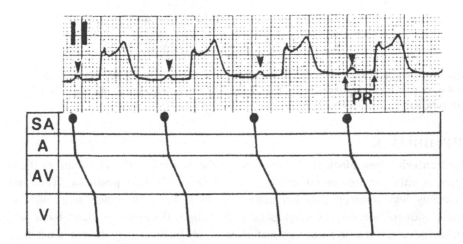

Fig. 7.8 **Fist degree AV block** in a 56-year-old woman with acute inferior myocardial infarction. Note: (1) "Hyperacute" phase of acute inferior myocardial infarction as reflected by elevated ST segment in lead II. (2) Prolonged PR interval of 0.28 sec. **The arrowheads in this and all subsequent figures indicate sinus P waves.**

Second degree AV block can be divided into **Mobitz type I (Wenckebach phenomenon), Mobitz type II, 2:1 and high grade AV block.** In Mobitz type I AV block, the ECG shows progressive prolongation of the PR interval, culminating in a dropped QRS complex, following which the whole sequence is repeated (Fig. 7.9). It may occur in highly trained athletes because of excess vagotonia and also in patients with acute inferior myocardial infarction or digitalis intoxication. The site of block is nearly always at the AV node, especially if the QRS is narrow and the prognosis is generally good.

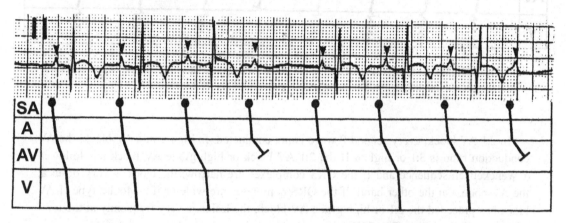

Fig. 7.9   Mobitz type I second degree AV block (Wenckebach phenomenon) in a patient with acute inferior myocardial infarction. Note: (1) Pathological Q wave, slightly elevated and coved ST segment, and T wave inversion in lead II reflecting the "resolution phase" of transmural inferior myocardial infarction. (2) Progressive prolongation of the PR interval culminating in non-conduction of the fourth P wave, following which the whole sequence is repeated.

In Mobitz type II AV block, the conducted beats show a constant PR interval and there is sudden failure of P wave conduction. The QRS complexes frequently show a bundle branch block pattern (Fig. 7.10). To qualify for the diagnosis of Mobitz type II AV block, the 2 sinus beats preceding and the 2 sinus beats following the blocked beat must be conducted. In Mobitz type II AV block, the lesion is very often at the bundle branches and the prognosis is considerably less favourable than Mobitz type I AV block, as it frequently proceeds to complete AV block and ventricular standstill. Cardiac pacing is indicated. The two common causes of Mobitz type II AV block are acute anterior myocardial infarction and degenerative disease of the conducting system.

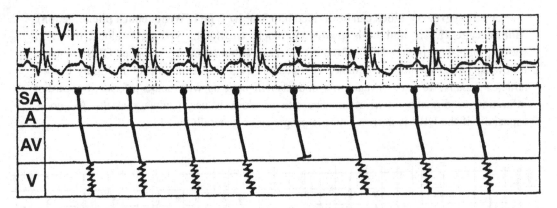

Fig. 7.10   Mobitz type II second degree AV block. Note: (1) Constant PR interval of 0.16 sec. (2) Sudden failure of conduction of the sixth P wave. (3) Wide QRS complexes.

In 2:1 AV block, every second P wave is not conducted. In high grade AV block, the AV conduction ratio is 3:1 or higher. If the 2:1 AV block or high grade AV block has followed a Wenckebach sequence and if the QRS complexes are narrow, the block is very often at the AV node. On the other hand, if the QRS complexes are wide or if a Mobitz type II AV block has preceded the 2:1 or high grade AV block, the lesion is very frequently at the level of the bundle branches (Fig. 7.11).

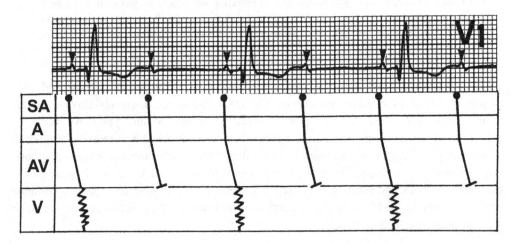

Fig. 7.11   2:1 second degree AV block. Note: (1) Every second P wave is blocked. (2) The conducted beats show a constant PR interval of 0.12 sec. (3) The QRS complexes show a complete right bundle branch block pattern. The site of the block is most likely at the level of the bundle branches.

In **third degree or complete AV block**, there is a failure of conduction of all the P waves. Third degree AV block may be due to a lesion at the AV node, the bundle of His or the bundle branches. In the last case, all 3 fascicles of the conducting system are blocked and the situation is essentially a **trifascicular block**.

If the block is at the AV node as in acute inferior myocardial infarction or congenital heart block, the escape pacemaker is situated at the AV junction and the QRS complexes are narrow. The ventricular rate, which is often around 40 to 60/min, can frequently be increased with intravenous atropine and syncope (**Stokes-Adams attacks**) are uncommon (Fig. 7.12). Cardiac pacing is usually unnecessary, except when the patient presents with heart failure or hypotension. On the other hand, in third degree (complete) AV block due to trifascicular block, the escape pacemaker is situated within the ventricles. The QRS complexes are widened and the ventricular rate, which is often very slow at around 30 to 40/min, usually cannot be increased with intravenous atropine. Stokes-Adams attacks are frequent and cardiac pacing is usually necessary (Figs. 7.13 and 7.14). Common causes of trifascicular block are acute anterior myocardial infarction, chronic degenerative disease of the conducting system, chronic ischaemic heart disease, post-cardiac surgery and acute myocarditis.

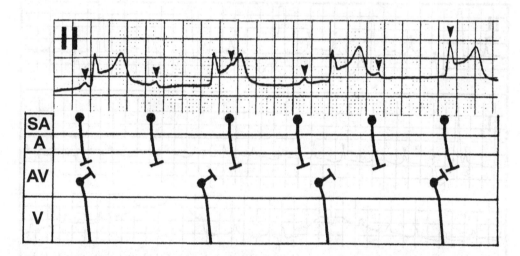

Fig. 7.12   **Third degree (complete) AV block** in acute inferior myocardial infarction. This ECG was recorded a few hours later than Fig. 7.8. Note: (1) Failure of conduction of all the P waves (2) Slow ventricular rate of 46/min (3) Narrow QRS complexes.

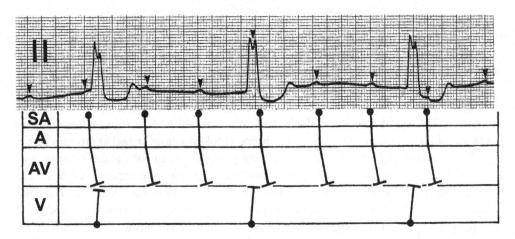

Fig. 7.13 ECG of a patient presenting with **third degree (complete) AV block**. The aetiology of the AV block most likely was idiopathic degeneration of both the bundle branches. Note: (1) Failure of conduction of all the P waves. (2) Very slow ventricular rate of 33/min. (3) Wide QRS complexes.

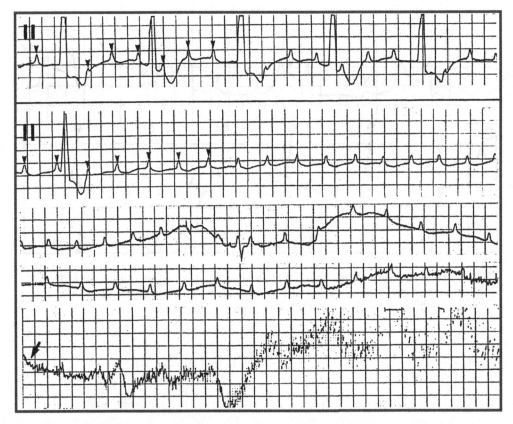

Fig. 7.14 ECG of a 16-year-old male with acute viral myocarditis. The ECG in the upper box shows **third degree (complete) AV block**, wide QRS complexes and a very slow ventricular rate of around 40/min. The ECG rhythm strips in the lower box are continuous and show third degree (complete) AV block and ventricular standstill resulting in syncope (Stokes-Adams attacks) and convulsons which have caused artifacts in the ECG (arrow).

In patients with third degree (complete) AV block who require cardiac pacing, either **temporary cardiac pacing** or **implantation of a permanent pacemaker** may be performed. If the complete AV block is temporary as most often is the case in acute inferior myocardial infarction, only temporary cardiac pacing is required. However, if it is chronic, which is frequently so in degenerative disease of the bundle branches, a permanent cardiac pacemaker will be required to be implanted. In patients with pacemakers employing the ventricular mode of pacing, the ECG shows spikes (due to ventricular pacemaker inpulses) which are immediately followed by wide QRS complexes (Fig. 7.15). In dual chamber pacing, each P wave is preceded by an atrial spike and this is followed, after a pre-set interval, by a ventricular spike which depolarizes the ventricles (Fig. 7.16).

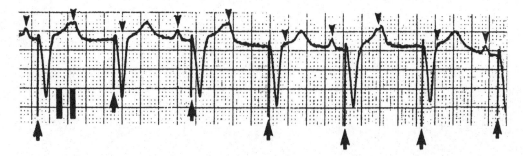

Fig. 7.15 Ventricular pacing in a patient with third degree (complete) AV block. Note: (1) Pacemaker spikes (arrows). (2) Wide QRS complex following each pacemaker spike because of non-simultaneous depolarization of the 2 ventricles. Arrowheads indicate sinus P waves.

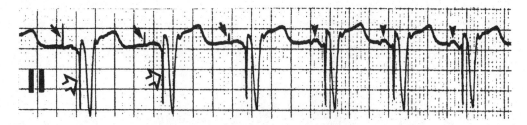

Fig. 7.16 Dual chamber pacing. Note atrial spikes (arrows) followed immediately by P waves in the first 3 beats. The next three P waves (arrowheads) are the patient's own sinus beats. After a pre-set interval of 0.20 sec, ventricular spikes (open arrows) are seen. They are followed immediately by wide QRS complexes reflecting non-simultaneous ventricular depolarization.

INDEX

A

Aberrant ventricular conduction   99
Accelerated idioventricular rhythm   110
Accelerated junctional rhythm   91
Acute coronary syndrome   16–38
    acute transmural myocardial infarction
      (STEMI)   17–31
    acute subendocardial myocardial
      infarction (NSTEMI)   32–37
    unstable angina   32–38
    Prinzmetal's angina   26, 27
Acute pericarditis   49
Acute pulmonary embolism   57
Adenosine   76, 87
Amiodarone   76, 112
Angina pectoris
    stable angina   38–41
Aortic regurgitation   55
Aortic stenosis   55
Arrhythmias, cardiac
    classification of   77
    diagnosis and treatment   73–76
Artifacts   71
Ashman's phenomenon   99
Athlete's heart syndrome   65
Atrial enlargement   56
    left atrial   52–56
    right atrial   54, 56
    bi-atrial   56
Atrial fibrillation   91–93
Atrial flutter   94–96
Atrial septal defect   119, 120
Atrioventricular (AV) block   122–126
    first degree   122
    second degree, Mobitz type I
      (Wenckebach phenomenon)   123

    second degree Mobitz type II   123
    second degree 2:1 and high grade AV
      block   124
    third degree or complete heart
      block   125, 126
Atrioventricular dissociation   109
Axis/axis deviation   6–8
    calculating   6–8
    normal   6–8
    left   6–8
    right   6–8
    "indeterminate"   7

B

Beta-blocker   76, 87
Bifasicular block   121
Brugada Syndrome   114
Bundle branch block
    complete and incomplete   118–120
    right   119
    left   118, 121
    right with left anterior hemiblock   120
    right with left posterior hemiblock   30

C

Cardiac arrest   112
Cardiomyopathy
    dilated   58, 59
    hypertrophic   59, 60
Carotid sinus massage   76, 87
Chronic obstructive lung disease   57
Compensatory pause
    complete   97
    incomplete   97
Complexes and segments   8, 9
Conducting system of the heart
    anatomy of   117

Coronary angiography   15, 27, 35
Coupling interval   101

D
De Winter T Wave   45
Dextrocardia   68
Digitalis
    effect   103
    intoxication   103–104

E
Early repolarization pattern   48
ECG, 12-lead   1–3
Einthoven triangle   5
Electrical cardioversion   76, 87, 110
Electrophysiology study   75

F
Fusion beat   107, 110

H
Heart rate, calculating   3–5
Hemiblock
    left anterior   121, 122
    left posterior   30, 121
Hexaxial reference system   6
Holter 24-hour monitor recording   75
Hyperkalaemia   63
Hypersensitive carotid sinus syndrome   80
Hypertension   53, 55
Hypocalcaemia   63, 64
Hypokalaemia   61, 62
Hypothermia   71

I
Idioventricular rhythm   113
Implantable cardioverter defibrillator   76, 113
Intracranial haemorrhage   61
Isoelectric line   9, 12

J
J point   9, 12
Junctional escape beat   81
Juvenile ECG pattern   63, 64

M
Mitral regurgitation   52, 55
Mitral stenosis   55, 56
Multifocal atrial tachycardia   83
Myocardial infarction, acute (STEMI)
    location of   19

    anterior   21–24
    inferior   21–24
    posterior   24
    right ventricular   24
    evolutionary pattern   18–20
    "hyperacute phase" of   19–21
    "fully evolved phase" of   20–22
    "resolution phase" of   19
    "chronic phase" of   20, 22
    Q wave   16
    non-Q wave   16
    with bundle branch block   30, 31
    reinfarction   31
Myxoedema   62

N
NSTEMI   32–37
    See acute coronary syndrome
Normal male pattern   47

O
Obesity   71
Oesophageal lead ECG   73, 74

P
Pacemaker
    temporary   127
    permanent   127
Percutaneous coronary intervention   28, 29
Pericardial effusion   50, 51
"P mitrale"   56
Poor R wave progression   19
"P pulmonale"   54, 56
Prinzmetal's angina   26, 27
Procaineamide   88
Pulmonary hypertension   55

Q
Q III   67
QRS alternans   50, 85, 90
QT (QTc) prolongation   13, 111, 112

R
Radiofrequency catheter ablation
    AV nodal reentrant tachycardia   87
    AV reentrant tachycardia   88
    atrial fibrillation   93
    atrial flutter   96
Reversal of right and left arm leads   69, 70
rSR'   118–120
Rule of bigeminy   101

S

S1, Q3, T3 pattern   57
Sick sinus syndrome
 sinoatrial block   79
 sinus arrest   80
 alternating bradycardia-tachycardia
  syndrome   80
Sinus arrhythmia   79
Sinus bradycardia   78
Sinus tachycardia   78
STEMI   17–31
 See acute coronary syndrome
Stokes-Adams attacks   126
ST segment depression   32–41, 44
 downsloping   32–39
 horizontal   32–39
 upsloping   33, 44
 reciprocal   20, 21
ST segment elevation   17–31, 44
Sudden cardiac death   112
Supraventricular ectopic beats   82–83
Supraventricular tachycardia   84–90
 AV nodal reentrant tachycardia   84
 AV reentrant tachycardia   85, 88
 atrial tachycardia   85
 with aberrant ventricular
  conduction   108
Syncope   75, 79

T

Takotsubo cardiomyopathy   70
thyrotoxicosis   71
Tilt-table test   75
"Torsades de pointes"   111, 112
Triaxial reference system   5
Trifascicular block   125, 126
Troponin   17, 32
T wave inversion   66
 giant T wave inversion   36–37

U

U wave inversion   41, 42

V

Valsalva manoeuvre   76
Ventricular aneurysm   20, 24
Ventricular asystole   113
Ventricular bigeminy   102
Ventricular ectopic beats   97–104
 Lown's grading system   99, 100
 uniform   98, 100
 multiform   98, 100
 "R on T"   101
 unifocal multiform   104
 in late diastole   116
Ventricular fibrillation   113, 114
Ventricular flutter   112
Ventricular hypertrophy   52–55
 left ventricular hypertrophy with strain
  pattern   53, 55
 right ventricular hypertrophy with
  strain pattern   54, 55
 biventricular hypertrophy   55
Ventricular tachycardia   105–112, 115
 monomorphic   105–109
 polymorphic   111, 112
 torsades de pointes   111, 112
 fasicular tachycardia   115
 bidirectional tachycardia   103
Verapamil   76, 87

W

Wandering pacemaker   81
Wellens Syndrome   44
Wolff-Parkinson-White (WPW)
 Syndrome   88–90
 accessory pathway
  (Bundle of Kent)   88
 pre-excitation   88
 delta wave   88
 Type A and B   88
 AV reentrant tachycardia   88
 atrial fibrillation   88–89
 Q waves   88

Printed in the United States
By Bookmasters